MW01031940

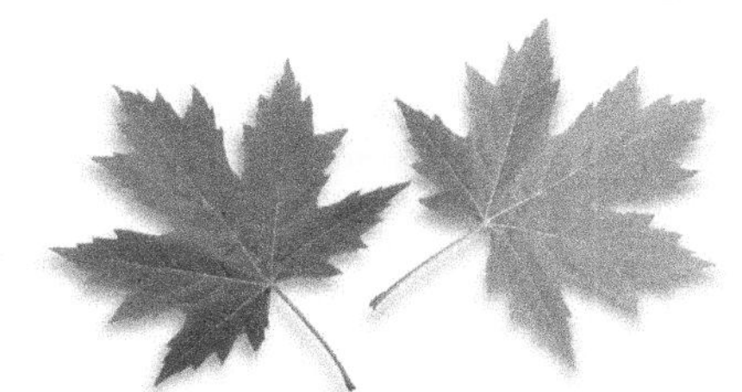

A PRACTICAL GUIDE FOR

Alzheimer's & Dementia CAREGIVERS

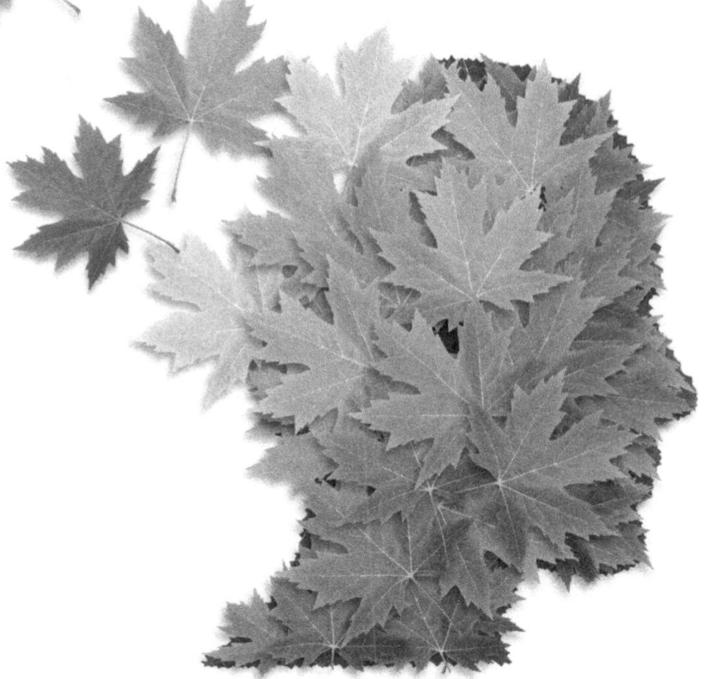

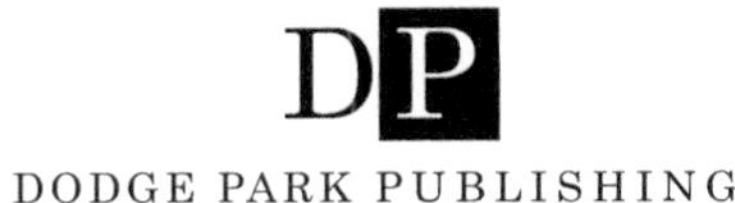

DODGE PARK PUBLISHING

A Practical Guide for
Alzheimer's & Dementia Caregivers
Micha Shalev

Paperback ISBN: 978-1-939288-42-4
eBook ISBN: 978-1-939288-49-3

Library of Congress Control Number: 2013957271

Edited by Karen V. Kibler

Indexed by Jean Jesensky, Endswell Indexing

www.dodgepark.com
Micha Shalev: M.Shalev@dodgepark.com

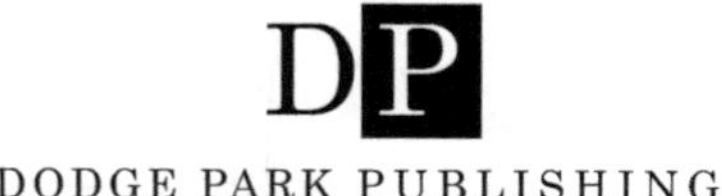

Published by Dodge Park Publishing
An Imprint of Wyatt-MacKenzie

Thank You

Special thanks to my wife, Sara Shalev, who supported me on this long road we have walked as professional caregivers, as well as with the unique challenges of writing this book. Without her work, assistance, advice, guidance, and support through the years, I would never have been able to accomplish all the milestones I have reached in my life. To my adorable and smart daughters, Karen and Maia, whom I love very much, thank you for being a part of my life, and providing much needed laughter, care, and joy, not only to me, but to the residents we all care for as one big family.

MICHA SHALEV

About the Author

Micha Shalev, MHA, CDP, CDCM, is the owner and administrator of Dodge Park Rest Home and The Adult Day Club at Dodge Park located at 101 Randolph Road in Worcester, MA. He has been involved with the geriatric field on both coasts for the past 27-plus years. He is an innovative long-term care administrator who always seeks new ways to improve resident care through resident center focus protocols. He is a graduate of the National Council of Certified Dementia Practitioners Program, as well as certified as a Dementia Care Manager, and has become a well-known speaker and trainer covering Alzheimer's and Dementia training topics for the past 27-plus years. The programs he created at Dodge Park Rest Home (and previously in Los Angeles, CA) are well known in the field of providing care for individuals diagnosed with dementia and Alzheimer's disease.

View more information online at http://www.dodgepark.com.

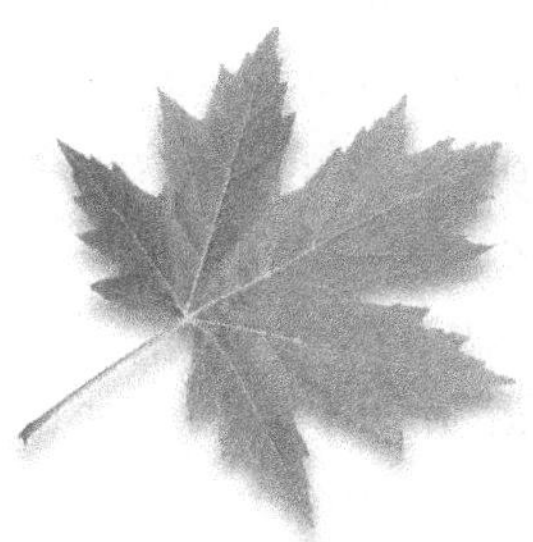

Introduction

In the challenging world of long-term care, there are exceptional people, who when times demand, will rise above the expectations of the norm and create a special climate of caring. This book is dedicated to all those wonderful, caring, and exceptional staff who assisted me in the past 27-plus years to deliver state-of-the-art resident center care for all the individuals we have cared for who suffer from dementia and Alzheimer's disease. Many of those individuals are no longer with us. May their souls rest in peace. I do hope and pray that their suffering will bring to light the urgent need for a new direction in dealing with this developing epidemic around the world, an epidemic that has ripped patients' personalities apart and left families heartbroken. There is a need for urgent collaboration among all the brightest minds around the world to try and come up with therapy, medications, and some sort of solution to deal with this unique disease.

My objective with this book is to create a practical guide through short articles that can assist caregivers in dealing with individuals diagnosed with dementia and/or Alzheimer's disease (AD) and the resulting challenges.

Dementia is often viewed as a disease of the mind, an illness that erases treasured memories but leaves the body intact. But as I have always stressed, dementia is a physical illness, too—a progressive, terminal disease that shuts down the body as it attacks the brain. The lack of understanding about the physical toll of dementia means that many patients near the end of life are subjected to aggressive treatments that would never be considered with other terminal illnesses.

I have tried to bring together as many articles as possible that I have authored and that have been published in various media; also included are some of the research projects of which I have been a part. There is a saying that personal observation of the very demanding world of caring for individuals diagnosed with dementia and/or AD is the best source of knowledge. I have to say that it is undoubtedly true. Over the years, I have revisited many protocols, care options, and staff training programs on a regular basis in an attempt to provide an environment that will support all the individuals for whom we provide care. I hope that you will all find this book to be easy to read, providing a simple guide to all caregivers—those who are just at the beginning of the road caring for a loved one, and those who are already well invested in providing care.

TABLE OF CONTENTS

PART I
Understanding Dementia

PART 3
Long-Term Care

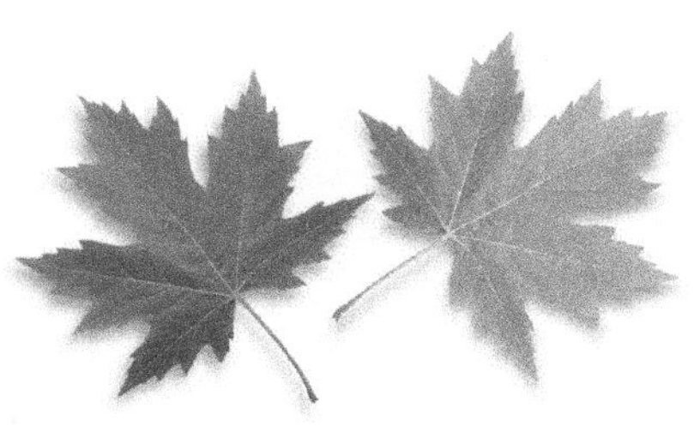

PART 1
Understanding Dementia

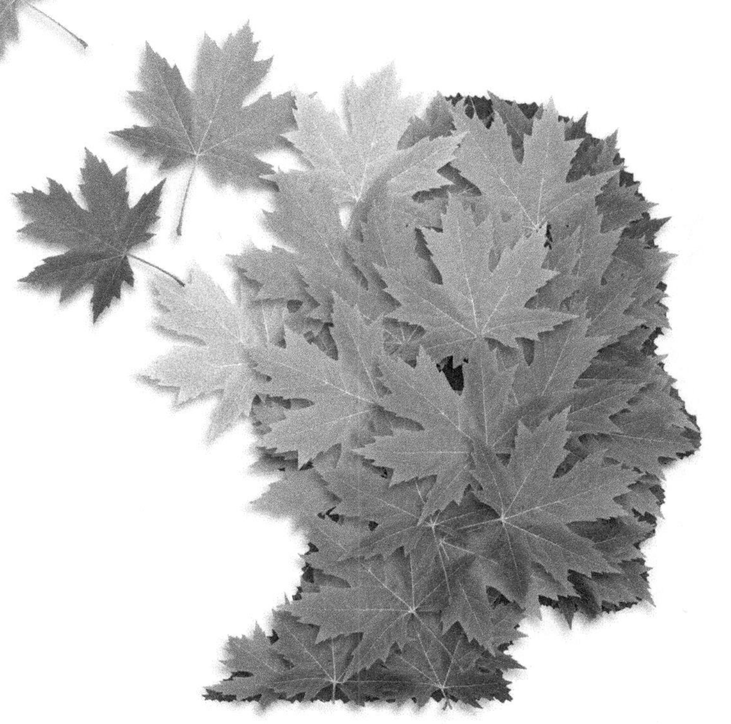

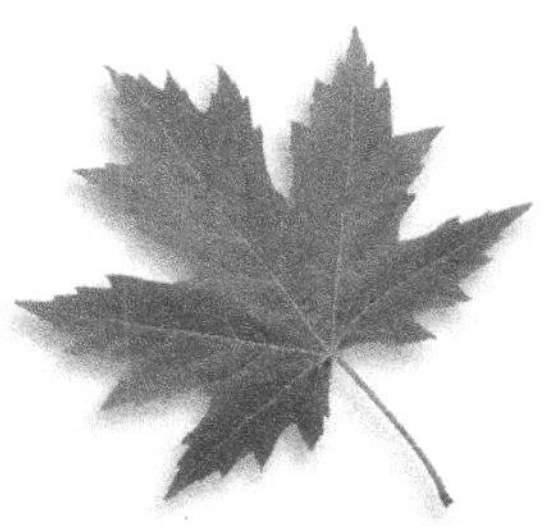

CHAPTER 1

Common Types of Dementia and Their Unique Characteristics

The term dementia is used broadly to describe a condition which is characterized by cognitive decline, but there are many different types of dementia. Although the disease is usually progressive, a proper and specific diagnosis can indicate treatments that will reverse the effects, and, at times, even lead to a cure by addressing the underlying cause. However, dementia caused by incurable conditions, such as Alzheimer's disease, is irreversible.

Dementia is caused by various diseases and conditions that result in damaged brain cells or connections between brain cells. When making a diagnosis of dementia, physicians commonly refer to the following criteria:

- Symptoms must include decline in memory *and* in at least one of the following cognitive abilities:

  Day-to-day memory

  Planning

Language

Attention

Visuospatial skills ("visuo" referring to eyesight and "spatial" referring to space or location), which give a person the ability to interpret objects and shapes.

- The decline in cognitive abilities must be severe enough to interfere with daily life.

Some individuals with memory problems and a decline in cognitive abilities have a condition called amnestic mild cognitive impairment (MCI) that often precedes Alzheimer's disease (AD). Individuals with MCI have more memory problems than normal for individuals their age, but their symptoms are not as severe as those seen in AD. Importantly, not all individuals with MCI develop AD.

In MCI, these symptoms will have been noticed by the individual and those who know them. If the person with MCI has taken cognitive function tests, their problems will be monitored and observed in test results over time. Any decline will be greater than the gradual decline that many people experience as part of normal, healthy aging. There may be minor problems with more demanding tasks, but generally not problems in everyday living (if there is a significant impact on everyday abilities, this may suggest dementia).

Memory loss and other cognitive problems can arise from many different causes. For some people diagnosed with MCI, memory loss will be the first sign of AD. For some of those with other cognitive problems, these will be the first signs of vascular dementia, frontotemporal dementia, or dementia with Lewy bodies.

It is important for a physician to determine the cause of memory loss or other dementia-like symptoms. Some symptoms can be reversed if they are caused by treatable conditions, such as depression, delirium, drug interaction, thyroid problems, excess use of alcohol, or certain vitamin deficiencies.

Vascular dementia

(also known as multi-infarct or post-stroke dementia or vascular cognitive impairment)

Vascular dementia is considered the second-most common type of dementia and is an umbrella term that describes impairments in cognitive function caused by problems in the blood vessels that feed the brain. In some cases, a blood vessel may be completely blocked, causing a stroke. Some strokes result in dementia while others don't. It depends on the severity of the stroke and the portion of the brain that is affected. Vascular dementia can also occur when blood vessels in the brain become narrowed, reducing the amount of blood flow to those sections of the brain.

Impairment is caused by decreased blood flow to parts of the brain, often due to a series of small strokes that block arteries. Symptoms often overlap with those of Alzheimer's, although memory may not be as seriously affected.

Mixed dementia

Mixed dementia is a condition in which abnormalities characteristic of more than one type of dementia occur simultaneously. Physicians may also call mixed dementia "Dementia-multifactorial."

In the most common form of mixed dementia, the abnormal protein deposits associated with AD coexist with blood vessel problems linked to vascular dementia. Alzheimer's changes to the brain also often coexist with Lewy bodies. In some cases, a person may have brain changes linked to all three conditions: AD, vascular dementia, and dementia with Lewy bodies.

Dementia with Lewy bodies

Dementia with Lewy bodies (DLB) is a type of progressive dementia that leads to a decline in thinking, reasoning, and independent function because of abnormal microscopic deposits that damage brain cells over time.

From my many years of observation, I strongly believe that dementia with Lewy bodies is among the most common causes of dementia after AD and vascular dementia. This belief is also supported by the Alzheimer's Association.

Parkinson's disease

Parkinson's disease (PD) belongs to a group of conditions called motor system disorders, which are the result of the loss of dopamine-producing brain cells. Some people with Parkinson's disease will develop dementia, usually after the age of 70 or as late as during the early 80s. The four primary symptoms of PD are tremor (trembling in hands, arms, legs, jaw, and face), rigidity (stiffness of the limbs and trunk), bradykinesia (slowness of movement), and postural instability (impaired balance and coordination). As these symptoms become more pronounced, patients may have difficulty walking, talking, or completing other simple tasks. PD usually affects people over the age of 50 (early stage). Early symptoms of PD are subtle and occur gradually. In some people the disease progresses more quickly than in others. As the disease progresses, the shaking, or tremor, which affects the majority of PD patients, may begin to interfere with daily activities. Other symptoms may include depression and other emotional changes, difficulty in swallowing, chewing, and speaking, urinary problems or constipation, skin problems, and sleep disruptions.

Frontotemporal dementia

Nerve cells in the front and side regions of the brain are especially affected. Typical symptoms include changes in personality and behavior, and difficulty with language. No distinguishing microscopic abnormality is linked to all cases. Pick's disease, characterized by Pick's bodies (nerve cells containing an abnormal accumulation of fibers made of the protein tau), is one type of frontotemporal dementia.

Creutzfeldt-Jakob disease

This is a rapidly fatal disorder that impairs memory and coordination and causes behavior changes. It is caused by the mis-folding of prion protein throughout the brain. Variant Creutzfeldt-Jakob disease (vCJD) is believed to be caused by consumption of products from cattle affected by mad cow disease, and is not related to classic CJD.

Normal pressure hydrocephalus

As with other manifestations of hydrocephalus, this dementia is caused by the buildup of fluid in the brain. Symptoms include difficulty walking, memory loss, and inability to control urination. The condition can sometimes be corrected with surgical installation of a shunt in the brain to drain excess fluid.

Alzheimer's disease

This is the most common type of dementia; it accounts for an estimated 60 to 80 percent of cases. Difficulty remembering names and recent events is often an early clinical symptom; apathy and depression are also often early symptoms. Later symptoms include impaired judgment, disorientation, confusion, behavior changes, and difficulty speaking, swallowing, and walking.

Hallmark abnormalities are deposits of the protein fragment beta-amyloid (plaques) and twisted strands of the protein tau (tangles).

Alzheimer's disease is the most common and most studied cause of dementia. Significant advances have been made since the first set of clinical criteria for AD were put forth in 1984 that are now captured in the new criteria for AD published in 2011. Key features in the updated criteria include recognition of a broad AD spectrum (from preclinical to mild cognitive impairment to AD dementia) and requirement of AD biomarkers for diagnosis. Correctly diagnosing dementia type is increasingly important in an era when potential disease-modifying agents are already, or are soon to be, marketed. The typical AD dementia syndrome has, at its core, an amnestic syndrome of the hippocampal type, followed by associated deficits in word-finding, spatial cognition, executive functions, and neuropsychiatric changes. Atypical presentations of AD have also been identified that are presumed to have a different disease course. It can be difficult to distinguish among the various dementia syndromes, given the overlap in many common clinical features across the dementias. The clinical difficulty in diagnosis may reflect the underlying pathology, as AD often co-occurs with other pathologies at autopsy, such as cerebrovascular disease or Lewy bodies. Neuropsychological evaluation has provided clinicians and researchers with profiles of cognitive strengths and weaknesses that help to define the dementias. As of yet, there is no single behavioral marker that can reliably distinguish AD from the other dementias. The combined investigation of cognitive and neurobehavioral symptoms coupled with imaging markers could provide a more accurate approach in the future for differentiating between AD and other major dementia syndromes.

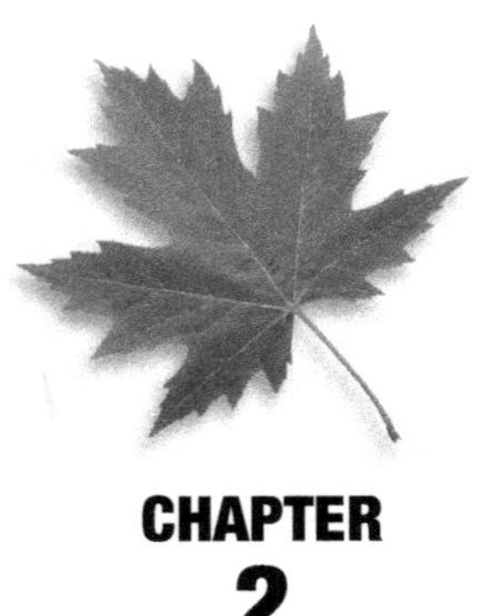

CHAPTER 2

What Is Alzheimer's Disease? What Causes Alzheimer's Disease?

Alzheimer's disease is a progressive neurologic disease of the brain leading to the irreversible loss of neurons and the loss of intellectual abilities, including memory and reasoning, which become severe enough to impede social or occupational functioning. Alzheimer's disease is also known as simply Alzheimer's, and Senile Dementia of the Alzheimer Type (SDAT).

At the annual meeting of the Radiological Society of North America in November 2012, researchers from the University of California reported that people who lead active lifestyles are more likely to slow down the progression of Alzheimer's disease, while active people who are Alzheimer's-free have a lower risk of developing the disease or any kind of dementia. Lifestyle factors that help ward off or slow down Alzheimer's include yard work, gardening, dancing, riding an exercise bike, and any type of aerobic exercise.

Why the name Alzheimer's disease?

Aloysius Alzheimer was a German neuropathologist and psychiatrist. He is credited with identifying the first published case of "presenile dementia" in 1906, which Dr. Emil Kraepelin later identified as Alzheimer's disease, naming it after his colleague.

In 1901, while he worked at the city mental asylum in Frankfurt am Main, Germany, Dr. Alzheimer had a 51-year-old patient, Mrs. Auguste Deter. The patient had distinct behavioral symptoms which did not fit any existing diagnoses—she had rapidly failing memory, disorientation and confusion, had trouble expressing her thoughts, and was suspicious about her family members and the hospital staff. Her symptoms progressed relentlessly. Dr. Alzheimer wrote that she once said to him, "I have lost myself."

Over the coming years, Auguste Deter would take up more and more of Dr. Alzheimer's time, to the point of almost becoming an obsession for him. Mrs. Deter died in 1906 and Dr. Alzheimer, who was working at Kraepelin's lab in Munich, had her patient records and brain sent to the lab in Munich.

Together with two Italian doctors, Dr. Alzheimer performed an autopsy. The autopsy revealed that her brain had shrunk dramatically, but there was no evidence of atherosclerosis (thickening and hardening of the walls of the arteries). He used a silver staining technique he had learned from a former colleague, Franz Nissl, which identified amyloid plaques and neurofibrillary tangles in the brain—two hallmarks of the disease.

Signs of Normal Change versus Early Alzheimer's Symptoms

Normal Aging	Early Alzheimer's Disease
Can't find the keys for the car or house.	Routinely place important items in odd places, such as keys in the fridge, wallet in the dishwasher.
Search for casual names and words.	Forget names of family members and common objects, or substitute words with inappropriate ones.
Briefly forget conversation details.	Frequently forget entire conversations that took place moments ago. Repeat questions multiple times.
Feel the cold more than when younger.	Dress without regard for the current weather: wear several skirts on a warm day, or shorts in a snowstorm; or wear clothes in improper order.
Can't find a recipe.	Can't follow recipe directions or simple instructions.
Forget to record a check.	Can no longer manage a checkbook, balance figures, solve problems, or think abstractly.
Cancel a date with friends.	Withdraw from usual interests and activities, sit in front of the TV for hours, sleep far more than usual.
Make an occasional wrong turn.	Get lost in familiar places, can't remember getting there or how to get home.
Feel occasionally sad.	Experience rapid mood swings, from tears to rage, for no discernible reason.

What are the symptoms of Alzheimer's disease?

Doctors say Alzheimer's disease can sometimes be tricky to diagnose because each patient has unique signs and symptoms. Several of the signs and symptoms present in Alzheimer's disease also exist in other conditions and diseases.

Alzheimer's disease is classified into several stages. Some doctors use a 7-stage framework, while others may use a 4-, 5- or 6-stage one. In my 27 years as a professional caregiver, I have come to use the 7-stage framework. It allows caregivers to better describe the stage of the disease and communicate the need to the family members as well as to the team of professionals in order to address the needs of the Alzheimer's patient.

What are the 7 stages of diagnostic framework?

A common framework for all classification systems includes: 1. Pre-dementia Stage; 2. Mild Alzheimer's Stage; 3. Moderate Alzheimer's Stage; 4. Severe Alzheimer's Stage. The details shown below are expanded to show the 7-stage framework.

STAGE 1: No Impairment

The person does not experience any memory problems. An interview with a medical professional does not show any evidence of symptoms of dementia.

STAGE 2: Minimal Impairment (Very Mild Cognitive Decline)

The person may feel as if he or she is having memory lapses—forgetting familiar words or the location of everyday objects. But no symptoms of dementia can be detected during a medical examination or by friends, family, or co-workers.

STAGE 3: Early Confusional (Mild Cognitive Decline); duration is two to seven years

The patient has begun to notice changes, such as:

- difficulty with remembering names when introduced to new people;
- noticeably greater difficulty performing tasks in social or work settings;
- forgetting material that one has just read;
- losing or misplacing valuable objects;
- decreasing ability to plan or organize.

STAGE 4: Moderate Cognitive Decline (Mild or Early Stage Alzheimer's disease); duration is about two years

At this point, a careful medical interview should be able to detect clear-cut symptoms in several areas:

- Forgetfulness of recent events;
- Impaired ability to perform challenging mental arithmetic—for example, counting backward from 100 by sevens;
- Greater difficulty performing complex tasks, such as planning a dinner for guests, paying bills or managing finances;
- Forgetfulness about one's own personal history;
- Becoming moody or withdrawn, especially in socially or mentally challenging situations.

STAGE 5: Moderately Severe Cognitive Decline (Moderate or Mid-stage Alzheimer's disease); duration is about 18 months

Gaps in memory and thinking are noticeable, and individuals begin to need help with day-to-day activities. At this stage, those with Alzheimer's may:

- Be unable to recall their own address or telephone number, or the high school or college from which they graduated;
- Become confused about where they are or what day it is;
- Have trouble with less challenging mental arithmetic, such as counting backward from 40 by 4s or from 20 by 2s;
- Need help choosing proper clothing for the season or the occasion;
- Still remember significant details about themselves and their family;

- Still require no assistance with eating or using the toilet.

STAGE 6: Severe Cognitive Decline (Moderately Severe Mid-stage Alzheimer's disease); duration is about two and a half years

Memory continues to worsen, personality changes may take place, and individuals need extensive help with daily activities. At this stage, individuals may:

- Lose awareness of recent experiences as well as of their surroundings;
- Remember their own name but have difficulty with their personal history;
- Distinguish familiar and unfamiliar faces but have trouble remembering the name of a spouse or caregiver;
- Need help dressing properly and may, without supervision, make mistakes such as putting pajamas over daytime clothes or shoes on the wrong feet;
- Experience major changes in sleep patterns—sleeping during the day and becoming restless at night;
- Need help handling details of toileting (for example, flushing the toilet, wiping, or disposing of tissue properly);
- Have increasingly frequent trouble controlling their bladder or bowels;
- Experience major personality and behavioral changes, including suspiciousness and delusions (such as believing that their caregiver is an impostor), or compulsive, repetitive behavior such as hand-wringing or tissue shredding;
- Tend to wander or become lost.

STAGE 7: Very Severe Cognitive Decline (Severe or Late-stage Alzheimer's disease); duration is one to two and a half years

In the final stage of this disease, individuals lose the ability to respond to their environment, to carry on a conversation and, eventually, to control movement. They may still say words or phrases.

At this stage, individuals need help with much of their daily personal care, including eating or using the toilet. They may also lose the ability to smile, to sit without support, and to hold their heads up. Reflexes become abnormal. Muscles grow rigid. Swallowing is impaired.

Life expectancy after the diagnosis

The primary reason that Alzheimer's disease shortens an individual's life expectancy is not usually the disease itself, but rather, the complications that result from it. As patients become less able to look after themselves, any illnesses they develop, such as an infection, are more likely to rapidly get worse. Caregivers will find it harder and harder to identify complications because the patient becomes progressively less able to tell if he/she is unwell, uncomfortable, or in pain. Pneumonia and pressure ulcers are examples of common complications which may lead to death for people with severe Alzheimer's disease.

Projected length of survival time following a diagnosis of Alzheimer's disease (AD) is important information for health planners, caregivers, patients, and their families. AD is associated with variable, but shortened life expectancy. Knowing the expected survival time may empower patients with AD and their families, but clinicians currently have limited predictive information. A better knowledge about prognosis in patients affected by AD and related disorders should be of paramount importance in order to improve care plans and assist in medical decisions; this is particularly important for patients in the moderate to severe stages of the disease. Life expectancy for patients with AD can vary between 3 and 10 years. Many studies have tried to identify predictive factors that can be of help to clinicians. The main predictor of life expectancy is the age of the patient at onset of disease. Therefore, caregivers, patients, and their families can plan on a median life span beyond onset according to the general guideline: as long as 7 to 10 years for patients whose conditions are diagnosed when they are in their 60s and early 70s; only about 3 years or less for patients whose conditions are diagnosed when they are in their 90s. Dementias with prominent psychiatric/behavioral manifestations and gait impairment have a faster progression compared to that of AD; however, the many variables that influence life expectancy make difficult the task of defining a prognosis at the bedside, and more studies are needed to assist clinicians in their daily routine with patients and caregivers.

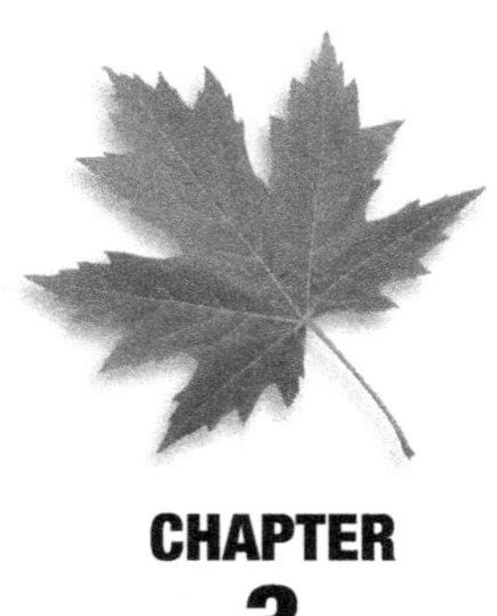

CHAPTER 3

Adjusting After the Diagnosis of Alzheimer's Disease

"Are you kidding me, I have what? It can't be true. It has to be a mistake." When you first receive a diagnosis of Alzheimer's, it can feel like the world is slipping away from you. It can be hard to move at all, much less stay positive and start making plans for the future that will make the later stages of the disease easier both for you and those around you. You may be really "angry." It's normal to have these feelings but the important thing is to find ways to cope, and continue to "have fun and laugh."

There are several methods and diagnostic tools to help determine fairly accurately whether an individual with memory problems has "possible Alzheimer's disease," "probable Alzheimer's disease," or some other memory or neurological problem.

"Possible Alzheimer's disease" is defined as a dementia that could be due to another condition. "Probable Alzheimer's disease" means no other causes for the symptoms can be found.

At this time, a definitive diagnosis of Alzheimer's disease (AD) can only be determined by an autopsy of the brain after death. However, at specialized centers, doctors can diagnose AD in a living person correctly up to 90 percent of the time.

A physician will diagnose Alzheimer's in a living person by:

- Asking questions about an individual's overall health, past medical history, ability to perform daily activities, and changes in behavior and personality;
- Conducting memory tests, and having the patient perform tasks such as problem solving, attention, counting, language skills, and other tasks related to brain functioning;
- Carrying out medical tests on blood, urine, or spinal fluid;
- Collecting information provided by family members or other caregivers about changes in a person's day-to-day function and behavior which may help in the diagnosis;
- Performing brain scans, such as magnetic resonance imaging (MRI), positron emission tomography (PET) scan, or a computed tomography (CT) scan.

A complete diagnostic workup for AD is lengthy and costly, and the process may take as long as a year or more before a final diagnosis is made. After the diagnosis is made, the family and patient may need considerable guidance and counseling. Family members often wonder whether they should tell their loved one of the diagnosis. While it is devastating to learn that your loved one has AD, it is frequently more stressful to be aware of the signs and symptoms and yet have no diagnosis for the problem. The family and the patient should agree regarding disclosure before the diagnosis is made, so that appropriate actions are taken. Not knowing always presents the risk of the family or friends finding out accidentally. Open and honest communications are best practice, but some families have their own reasons for choosing a different path. Families often look to healthcare professionals for guidance, and it is important for those professionals to then respect the decisions of the family; however, physicians are advised to disclose the diagnosis to their patients.

The American Psychiatric Association recommends advising AD patients and their families of the need for financial and legal planning due to the patient's eventual incapacity (e.g., power of attorney for medical and financial decisions, an up-to-date will, and the cost of long-term care).

In the long run, most people find that the best thing to do with an Alzheimer's diagnosis is to stay as proactive as possible, and to try to keep a sense of humor, especially when they're having a bad day. Most patients will have good days and bad days. If you're having a bad day, just hold on, because a good day will come along soon.

Finding support

Many resources and support options are available to assist you or your loved one in dealing with the diagnosis of AD. You can:

- Contact the Alzheimer's Association 24/7 Helpline at 1-800-272-3900. They can provide information, referrals, and care consultation.
- Join the Alzheimer's online community at https://www.alzconnected.org/ and share your experiences with others who know what you are going through.

- See *Living with Alzheimer's* (http://www.alz.org/living_with_alzheimers_4521.asp) for tips in how to cope with the changes you may be experiencing.
- Go to the Alzheimer's free online tool, *Alzheimer's Navigator*, (https://www.alzheimersnavigator.org/) to receive a customized action plan and step-by-step guidance on topics including driving and home safety.
- Reach out to your local Alzheimer's Association (map of US local chapters at http://www.alz.org/apps/findus.asp) which offers programs and services tailored to your needs and available community resources.

What is an Alzheimer's/dementia support group?

Caring for someone with AD impacts every aspect of daily life. As Alzheimer's patients lose one ability after another, caregivers face tests of stamina, problem solving, and resiliency. During this long and difficult journey, communication diminishes and rewards decrease; without strong support, caretakers face challenges to their own well-being.

Maintaining emotional and physical fitness is crucial. Preparing and protecting yourself, working to understand your loved one's experience, and embracing help from others can minimize the hazards and enhance the joys of your caregiving experience.

The purpose of an Alzheimer's support group is to offer individuals support and information that is specific to dementia. Some Alzheimer's Association chapters have specialized support groups, such as: early stage groups, groups for adolescents, male care partners, adult children caring for a parent, and care partners dealing with late stage issues.

An Alzheimer's Association-affiliated support group can be made up of care partners, family members, and loved ones of those with AD or a related dementia. Although these people begin as strangers, they quickly become friends and, in a sense, a family. The support group leader may be a community member and/or a health care professional. The meeting may focus on emotional support and sharing experiences, or it may focus on education, with experts speaking on topics such as legal issues, nutrition, caregiving techniques, and community resources.

The number of participants will vary in some cases, depending on the format. For instance, educational groups are usually larger. However, the ideal size for a support group is 6 to 24 members.

Support groups that are sponsored by the Alzheimer's Association are open to the public and free of charge. These support groups depend on their affiliated chapters to provide resources such as literature, updates on legislation and research, and newsletters. Alzheimer's Association chapters serve larger areas than do the support groups, and they provide resources to the community as well.

Alzheimer's Association support groups encourage members to share information, give and receive mutual support, and exchange coping skills with one another. Support group members share practical suggestions for caring based on their caregiving experiences. Caring for an individual with dementia requires different techniques than those needed to care for someone who is not cognitively impaired.

Experienced care partners have found that some methods of providing care, ideas that may not be found in books or articles, can make caregiving easier. Sharing such ideas in a support group can prevent care partners from having to "re-invent the wheel."

Attending a support group is often difficult at first. It takes time to feel comfortable sharing your problems with people you do not know. However, the experience of many individuals is that once they open up, they find that their problems are not so different from those of other support group members. Suddenly, the people they are sharing with are not strangers at all, and by sharing with others in the same situation they feel less alone.

If you are having difficulty talking to family or friends about your feelings, you may find that it is easier to express yourself in a support group, where you can be honest with others who are facing similar problems. Through participation in a support group, you will be better prepared, and perhaps feel less devastated as your loved one's condition becomes worse. You may also be able to find some hope, from seeing that others who have been providing care longer than you, have survived the caregiving experience.

Remember that if you attend a group(s) and it doesn't feel right for you, you can always try another group.

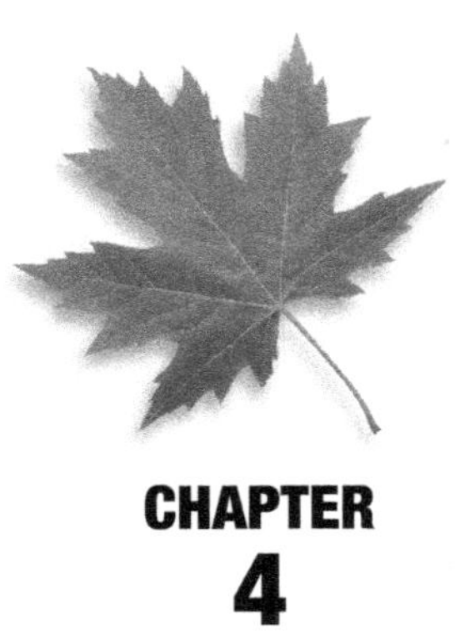

CHAPTER 4

One Likely Cause of Memory Impairment That Is Rarely Suspected

When life's challenges include memory loss or dementia, your perceptions, relationships, and priorities inevitably shift. Changes to our sleep patterns naturally occur with aging, but scientists are finding links between changes to sleep and senior memory impairment, cognitive decline, and even dementia.

When we get older, we begin to forget things. That's the common wisdom anyway, and it's not far from the truth. It's long been known that sleep plays a strong role in memory consolidation; but now, research is showing that age-related changes to the sleeping brain disrupt the normal pathways to memory formation, leading to that form of forgetfulness we associate with growing older. Some studies are even showing an increased risk of cognitive impairment and/or dementia linked with disrupted sleep patterns: (http://www.aplaceformom.com/-blog/2013-03-7-sleepproblems-senior-health-caregivers/).

One of the exciting recent discoveries scientists have made in the area of sleep and memory research is that there is a link between poor sleep and memory loss in the aging brain. Neuroscientists at the University of California, Berkeley, reported their findings in a recent study that compared memory retention in groups of younger adults and older adults. Conducted in 2012 and published in Nature Neuroscience, the study found that in elderly people, age-related deterioration of the prefrontal cortex region of the brain was associated with a failure to achieve the kind of deep, slow-wave sleep that helps the brain consolidate memories and information.

Another recent study, conducted by Elizabeth Devore, from the Brigham and Women's Hospital in Boston, Massachusetts looked at 15,000 women, aged 70 or older, over a period of five years. The women had all undergone a routine test to check their attention, concentration, and memory span. It was found that those who usually slept for seven hours each night performed much better than those who slept less than five hours or more than nine. According to a spokesperson for the Alzheimer Society who reviewed the study, "A good night's sleep is one of the pleasures of life, but, once again, the study conducted by Brigham and Women's Hospital in Boston strongly suggests that the quality and duration of sleep has been also linked to people's cognitive health." Too much sleep can be an issue as well. It is far too early to conclude that lack of sleep plays a causal role in dementia, but there is certainly compelling evidence in past years that getting enough quality sleep is an essential preventative health measure—which means that those at mid-life and older who are experiencing sleep problems should try to solve them (easier said than done, I realize).

Though it may seem there is nothing we can do about the inevitable changes that take place in our brains as we age, there is a hopeful and positive outcome of recent research. The researchers' findings may help future studies pinpoint new treatment angles for age-related memory loss. In fact, scientists are already designing studies to determine whether enhancing sleep in older adults can improve their overnight memory retention.

There is another, more serious reason to tackle the problem of poor sleep in seniors: the risk of developing cognitive impairment or dementia later in life. Not only do people get less deep sleep as they get older, but also (according to the National Institutes of Health), they are more likely to experience disruptions to their sleep schedule, suffer from insomnia or sleep apnea, or develop movement disorders such as restless legs syndrome, that keep them from getting a good night's sleep. Scientists are now finding that some of these sleep disruptions are associated with impaired cognition and, in some cases, the later onset of dementia.

In the end, however, it is important to remember that there is not a simple cause-and-effect relationship between sleep and dementia risk, or sleep and memory loss. The interactions between sleep, brain changes, and cognitive impairment are complex, and just as there are many factors that cause changes in sleep as our loved ones get older, there are numerous causes for age-related mental decline. Getting a good night's sleep is just one piece of the puzzle.

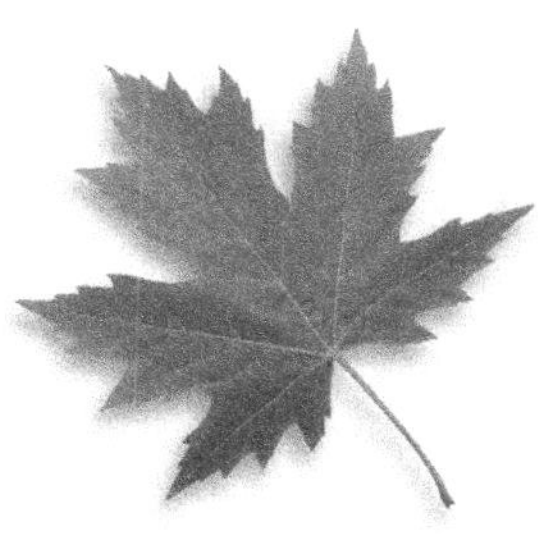

CHAPTER 5

Sleep Problems in the Elderly With Dementia

Sleep disorders are commonly underdiagnosed and are a significant source of concern in the geriatric population.

Age alone does not cause sleep problems. Disturbed sleep, waking up tired every day, and other symptoms of insomnia are not a normal part of aging. Instead, poor sleep habits, untreated sleep disorders, medications, or medical problems can contribute to sleeplessness. This section will help you understand the causes of sleep problems and provide tips to help you or your patient sleep well with more benefit.

In addition to affecting quality of life (including excessive daytime sedation, and physical, psychological, or cognitive problems affecting overall health of the resident), sleep disorders have been implicated with an increased mortality rate. Unfortunately, the number of medications increases with age, which in itself can lead to more morbidity, mortality, and side effects such as falls, cognitive impairment, financial stressors, and even sleep disturbances. In elderly patients diagnosed with dementia, treating insomnia can improve the overall health of the resident, but care must be taken when medications are used to treat this particular population.

Resident education about age-related changes in sleep can alter residents' expectations. An example is a situation in which, as a result of education, a resident realizes that an occasional sleepless night does not indicate a health problem.

Residents should be encouraged to improve sleep hygiene and use behavioral interventions. For example, to improve sleep hygiene, residents are reminded not to consume stimulants (e.g., caffeine) for several hours before bedtime.

Behavioral interventions include sleep restriction therapy (limiting the time spent in bed and minimizing daytime napping). This therapy increases sleep efficiency; it may deprive residents of some sleep, but usually only initially.

Residents are instructed to awaken at the same time each morning; they determine when to go to bed based on their usual total number of nightly sleep hours, estimated by using a sleep diary. The time spent in bed is gradually increased as sleep efficiency increases.

Bright light therapy may help residents with an advanced or a delayed sleep phase. In sunny climates, outdoor bright light exposure may work just as well. A clinician should review all drugs that residents are taking to check whether any may induce photosensitivity and should determine whether residents have other disorders that may be exacerbated by this therapy.

Until recently, poor sleep patterns in people with dementia was taken as an irreversible aspect of the disease. Today, however, studies are increasingly showing that sleep quality in people with dementia can indeed be improved, and, consequently, symptoms of poor sleep, such as sundowning, insomnia, and excessive daytime sleepiness, can be diminished.

Improved sleep means an improved quality of life for a person with dementia through increased alertness, decreased sleepiness, and reduction in behavioral problems. These beneficial consequences have a positive impact on a caregiver's quality of life and the quality of care the caregiver is able to give. Normally, a caregiver's own sleep quality begins to suffer as the caregiver deals with a wandering or belligerent person. A moment of inattentiveness on a tired caregiver's part can potentially allow the person with dementia to get into dangerous situations. Persistent poor sleep quality can cause the caregiver to suffer negative mood changes, such as depression, anger, hopelessness, etc., which in turn can negatively impact the quality of care the caregiver is able to provide to someone with dementia. Poor sleep quality and its impact on the caregiver may be the most common factor leading caretakers to institutionalize a person with dementia. However, as the McCurry study (*Current Psychiatry Reports* 2009, 11[1]:20) suggests, improving sleep quality in a person with dementia may delay having to place the person in an institutional setting and may improve quality of life, not only that of the person with dementia, but also that of the caregivers.

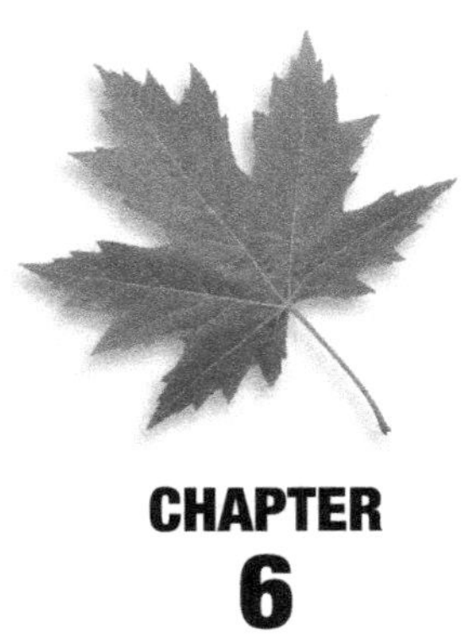

CHAPTER 6

Troubling Behavior in People With Dementia

Dementia is not an inevitable consequence of aging, but the risk of dementia increases sharply with advancing age and prevalence is expected to increase dramatically over the coming decades. Dementia features an alteration of memory and at least one other cognitive disorder such as aphasia, apraxia, or a disturbance in executive functioning. Though various etiologies are related to dementia, such as strokes, head trauma, Parkinson's disease, and substance abuse, Alzheimer's disease is considered the most widespread form of all senile dementias, representing more than half of all cases. The onset of dementia of the Alzheimer's type is gradual and involves continuing cognitive decline.

In addition to cognitive symptoms, persons with dementia often present behavioral and psychological symptoms which may increase their suffering, be difficult to manage by caregivers, and precipitate institutionalization. Behavioral symptoms of dementia include sundowning, wandering, agitation, screaming, and hitting, while psychological symptoms include hallucinations, delusions, and depression. Between 50 and 90 percent of dementia patients present behavioral or psychological symptoms.

Sundowning

Some people with Alzheimer's disease symptoms seem to grow worse in the late afternoon or evening. They become particularly agitated and have trouble going to bed and staying asleep. Experts believe this behavior, commonly called sundowning, is caused by a combination of exhaustion and changes in the person's biological clock that confuse day and night, possibly leaving them unable or unwilling to cope with minimal demands.

Sundowning, or "sundown syndrome," describes the behavioral symptoms such as confusion and agitation that can be observed at the end of the day and that often continue into the night.

Sundowning is not a disease, but is a set of symptoms often associated with cognitive and affective disorders common in older adults, similar to delirium, dementia, and depression.

Sundowning in demented individuals, as a distinct clinical phenomenon, is still open to debate in terms of clear definition, etiology, operationalized parameters, validity of clinical construct, and interventions. A variety of treatment options have been found to be helpful to ameliorate the neuropsychiatric symptoms associated with this phenomenon, including some medications.

Symptoms of sundowning may include:

- "Benign" visual hallucinations (as opposed to frightening hallucinations that occur in psychotic patients; for example, one may see a visitor no one else can see)
- Disorientation/confusion
- Agitation
- Disinhibition
- Paranoia
- Pacing aimlessly and continuously

The direct cause of sundowning is unknown, but circadian rhythm is thought to be related as it influences physiological processes that regulate body functions and behavior. Disruptions in circadian rhythm may cause irregular changes in physiological processes such as core body temperature and hormonal secretions. Other factors, such as fatigue, low lighting, and shadows, may contribute to sundowning.

Social and environmental interventions may help to mitigate sundowning symptoms. Attention should be given to lighting appropriate to the time of day and sleep needs, window shades that may be open or closed, structured meal times, suitable visitors and visiting hours, and morning and bedtime routines. A midafternoon nap or quiet time should be encouraged. Noise and other sensory stimulation should be limited before bedtime. And in an unfamiliar setting such as a hospital, familiar items such as photographs may help reduce agitation and confusion.

Tips for managing sundowning in the context of home care:

- Try to increase the patient's activity during the daytime. Provide activities that encourage use of excess physical energy, such as walking in a familiar, secure environment, exercise classes, yoga, stretching, gardening, and sweeping.
- Watch out for foods that can increase insomnia, particularly in someone sensitive to it. These include sugar, caffeine, and some types of junk food. Eliminate such foods and beverages, or restrict to the early hours of the day.
- Plan to serve frequent small meals throughout the day, including a light meal, such as half a sandwich, before bedtime.
- Plan the day so that afternoon and evening hours are quiet and calm but not boring or empty. Quiet, structured activity helps. Decrease noise, clutter, and activity that can add to confusion and anxiety.
- Turning on lights well before sunset and closing the curtains at dusk will minimize shadows and may help diminish confusion. Make sure there are night-lights in the person's room, hallway, and bathroom.
- Do not restrain the individual, which may provoke a catastrophic reaction. Do not argue or rationalize with the patient; instead, reassure.
- Prolonged pacing expends tremendous energy. The residents may lose weight. Check with a nurse or physician. Prolonged pacing may also cause loss of fluid. This can be serious if dehydration leads to physical complications and increased confusion. Distract when possible with another

activity. Provide articles or activities which provide comfort or security for the individual, such as a favorite blanket or doll; soothing, familiar music; or a quiet task of "folding towels."

- Also, be sure that the house is safe. Use gates to block off stairs, lock the kitchen door, and put away dangerous items. If nothing helps, you may want to talk to the doctor about medication to help an agitated person relax and sleep. Be aware that sleeping pills and tranquilizers may solve one problem and create another, such as sleeping at night but being more confused the next day.
- It is essential that you, the caregiver, get enough sleep. If your loved one's nighttime activity keeps you awake, consider asking a friend or relative, or hiring someone, to take a turn so that you can get a good night's sleep. Catnaps during the day might also help.

Tips for managing sundowning in the context of long-term facility care:

- Try to increase the patient's activity during the daytime. Provide activities that encourage use of excess physical energy, such as walking in a familiar, secure environment, exercise classes, yoga, stretching, gardening, and sweeping.
- Know if your patient is sensitive to foods that can induce insomnia, such as sugar, caffeine and some types of junk food, and ask that the facility eliminate such foods and beverages, or restrict to the early hours of the day.
- Find out if the facility offers frequent small meals throughout the day, including a light meal, such as half a sandwich, before bedtime.

- Be sure that the facility provides structure so that the resident feels safe and knows what is expected. Decreased noise, clutter, and activity will help to avoid confusion and anxiety.
- Turning on lights well before sunset and closing the curtains at dusk will minimize shadows and may help diminish confusion. Make sure there are night-lights in the person's room and bathroom.
- Ask that the staff not restrain the individual, which may provoke a catastrophic reaction. Ask that the staff not argue or rationalize with the patient; instead, they should reassure.
- Prolonged pacing expends tremendous energy. The residents may lose weight. Check with a nurse or physician. Prolonged pacing may also cause loss of fluid. This can be serious if dehydration leads to physical complications and increased confusion. Distract when possible with another activity. Provide the facility with articles or activities which provide comfort or security for the individual, such as a favorite blanket or doll; a means of listening to soothing, familiar music; or provide for a quiet task of "folding towels" that can be offered to the patient by the facility staff.
- Also, be sure that the facility is safe. Stairs should be blocked off with gates and doors to other areas locked. If nothing helps, consult with the patient's doctor about medication to help your patient relax and sleep. Be aware that sleeping pills and tranquilizers may solve one problem and create another, such as sleeping at night but being more confused the next day.

Agitation

The term "agitation" is very often used in reference to behavioral symptoms associated with dementia. Agitation was originally defined as any inappropriate verbal, vocal, or motor activity which, according to an outside observer, does not result directly from the needs or the confusion of the agitated person. Behavior which constitutes agitation can be broadly classified as aggressive versus non-aggressive and physical versus verbal. A factor analysis of a measure of agitation used with nursing home residents produced three factors which make it possible to distinguish various forms of agitation: aggressive behavior (AB, e.g., hitting), non-aggressive physical behavior (NAPB, e.g., pacing), and verbally agitated behavior (VAB, e.g., complaining).

The specific determinants of agitation remain unclear. Predisposing factors may include gender, personality, poor health, functional impairment of activities of daily living, as well as cognitive and neurological deterioration. Other factors may precipitate the occurrence of agitation and include the characteristics of the physical and social environment (e.g., too much noise, not enough social interaction) as well as physical needs such as hunger, thirst, and discomfort. Some of these variables, such as gender, the severity of cognitive impairment, and the level of dependence in performing activities of daily living, are well documented in the literature in terms of their relationship with different types of agitation. For example, males are more likely to be aggressive than females.

Learning to communicate to calm the agitation

People with dementia often find it hard to remember the meaning of words or to think of the words they want to say.

During the late phases of the illness, people with dementia may communicate mainly by gestures and expressions. The following suggestions may help you communicate with a person who has dementia and is agitated:

- If you are about to lose your temper, try "counting to ten," remembering that the person has a disease and is not deliberately trying to make things difficult for you.
- Try and talk about feelings rather than arguing over facts.
- Identify yourself by name and call the person by name. Approach the person slowly from the front and give him or her time to become accustomed to your presence.
- Try to talk in a quiet place without too much background noise.
- Speak slowly and distinctly. Use familiar words and short sentences.
- Keep things positive.
- Use gestures, visual cues, and verbal prompts to help.

Wandering

People suffering from dementia display many common behavioral traits, and one of the hardest to manage and understand is wandering. Wandering may be a response to restlessness, agitation, fear, boredom, or physical discomfort. It may be a continued expression of a life-long habit of walking originally in a work situation or leisure-time pursuit. Wandering, in some cases, may be viewed as a positive activity when contained in a hazard-free environment.

There are a number of reasons that people with Alzheimer's wander away and get lost. Often they have forgotten where they are or they decided to do something and then got lost when they forgot what it was they were trying to achieve. This is not always the case, however, as wandering may instead be a sign of distress or illness.

We are all wanderers, of course, to varying degrees. And it is no surprise that when our memories begin to slip, when our days fade, when our lives become broth-thin, and we walk around as living ghosts of the vibrant people we once were, we start looking for a way out, an exit. Dementia-driven wandering can seem random to others, but it can be the result of boredom, curiosity, or just a general desire to get up and go. Caregivers tell stories of patients wanting to go home, even when they are home.

The literature of wandering—Homer's *Odysseus*, Coleridge's *Ancient Mariner*, Steinbeck's *Dust Bowl* families, *Star Trek*'s questing starships, for instance—fills shelves and shelves. "One wanders through life as if wandering through a field in the dark of night," is an excerpt from a quote by Lemony Snicket, who is an American novelist.

Some of the problems resulting from the patient wandering include: other patients and caregivers are annoyed by the person who is wandering around; the patient/resident may try to leave the area unattended; the patient becomes suspicious, disoriented, and possibly hallucinates.

Discovering the triggers for wandering is not always easy, but recognizing them can provide insights to dealing with the behavior. Possibilities include:

• Stress and anxiety

Although stress and anxiety are a normal and unavoidable aspect of life, the way we cope will depend on a number of things. When you have dementia, wandering away may be one way to express stress and/or anxiety. The inability to think clearly through the steps of an action prior to acting has a major impact on expression of uncomfortable feelings.

• Restlessness and agitation

Restlessness and agitation in Alzheimer's can cause many different types of behavior, and wandering is only one of them.

• Confusion, related to time and place

• A desire to fulfill former obligations

This impulse can reflect a variety of prior activities: going to work, going to the subway, caring for a husband or child, meeting family and friends.

• Medication, medication side effects

Drugs used to treat medical illness and conditions can sometimes result in unwanted side effects. An example of this is medications used to treat agitation. Diazepam can result in lessened anxiety but increase disinhibited behavior. Other drugs can cause agitation, or can make someone feel physically uncomfortable. Wandering may result.

- **An inability to recognize the familiar**

  Not being able to recognize familiar people, places, and objects can cause the patient to feel fear, panic, or simply the desire to go and find some place that they do recognize.

- **Fear arising from the misinterpretation of sights and sounds**

  Some people with dementia may run away in order to get away if they are frightened by something. This may be a result of misinterpreting something going on in their environment.

To address the wandering, try attending to the triggers listed above, such as boredom, worry, hunger, pain, or the need to use a bathroom. Help the patient make sense of his environment, which may reduce feelings of anxiety and the concomitant "searching." Label clearly all areas such as bathrooms, dining areas, and the patient's room (at home or in a facility). Family members may recognize factors in the patient's history that have ignited the need to wander, such as a job that involved walking: mail carrier, meter reader, factory supervisor, etc. Observe the patient's patterns and time of wandering. Are there triggering incidents related to staff or caregiver behavior which could be avoided?

As the number of Alzheimer's patients grows, organizations and companies are developing potentially helpful technologies. LoJack, the stolen-automobile recovery company, offers a SafetyNet bracelet that allows people to keep track of dementia-driven wanderers via radio signals. A shoe company, Aetrex Worldwide, and a firm that makes global positioning devices, GTX Corporation, have created shoes containing GPS technology for wanderers to wear. But there are simple actions that can also help: provide a medical alert bracelet to inform responders who find a patient wandering alone and away from the home; keep a photo and a piece of unwashed clothing of the patient's in a plastic bag to assist in the search if the patient wanders from the home or facility.

Wandering is a potentially life-threatening danger that can cause acute stress for both the patient and the patient's caregivers. It is important to recognize the confusion and help him or her refocus on real-life tasks.

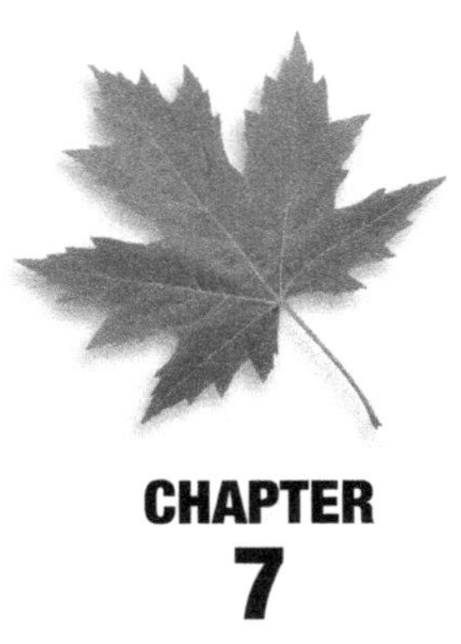

CHAPTER 7

Alzheimer's Disease and Religious Belief

The United States is currently experiencing the early stages of what is expected to be an epidemic of Alzheimer's disease. It is predicted that the current number of cases of Alzheimer's disease will double by 2020, and double again by 2040. Some unfortunate individuals are born with genes that strongly predispose them to developing Alzheimer's and/or dementia. However, this is true for only a minority of people. The familial, early onset form of Alzheimer's and/or dementia, which is so strongly linked to genetic abnormalities, is responsible for only about five percent of all cases of this illness. There is compelling evidence that the rest of us can escape, or at least postpone or diminish, the severity of Alzheimer's by improving our diets and maintaining a healthier lifestyle. In most cases, it appears Alzheimer's and other forms of dementia can be avoided.

An underappreciated, but validated belief within the field of long-term care, is that a good education, challenging your mind, maintaining friendships, and staying socially active, can also help reduce the risk of developing Alzheimer's and/or dementia in later life. A new report in the American Medical Association Journal, Archives of General Psychiatry, now complements those findings in showing that simply having a sense of purpose in life can help to reduce this risk.

This study suggests that people who say their lives have a purpose are less likely to develop Alzheimer's disease or its precursor, mild cognitive impairment. Purpose—which the researchers define as "a psychological tendency to derive meaning from life's experiences and to possess a sense of intentionality and goal directedness that guides behavior"—has long been thought to protect against adverse health outcomes. Purposeful living was recently reported to be associated with longevity as well. But there was little information on the association of purpose with Alzheimer's disease.

As one's words and cognitive ability fade, symbols of faith can still elicit responses. The appearance of a cross or a Star of David, or holding a Bible, a prayer book, or a rosary, can spark emotions that connect to religious activities of the past. Dr. David Wentroble, who is the director of pastoral care at Nyack Hospital in Nyack, New York, suggests that making a *reminiscence packet* for your loved one with Alzheimer's or dementia will help him/her to better deal with the overall medical problems.

You may want to create a reminiscence packet that you can carry and bring along on your visits.

Below are some ideas to help you develop a meaningful reminiscence packet for your loved one. Suggestions vary based on different faith traditions:

Catholic: Crucifix, rosary, scapular, sacred heart badge, or a statue of Mary; prayer cards for The Lord's Prayer, 23rd Psalm, Ten Commandments, Apostle's Creed, Hail Mary, Magnificat, mysteries of the Holy Rosary, and prayer to the Sacred Heart.

Protestant: Bible, cross, or a traditional picture of Jesus; prayer cards for The Lord's Prayer, 23rd Psalm, Ten Commandments, and Numbers 6: 24-26.

Jewish: Prayer book, yarmulkes, tallit, tefillin, mezuzah, Star of David, Kiddush cup, and candlesticks.

Having your loved one hold and touch such familiar objects, or listen to a familiar prayer or song, can be a unique way of communicating when words are fading. This can be very reassuring to someone with Alzheimer's. The memories of comforting religious activities can long outlast orientation to current time and place.

One of my dearest clients once told me: "I pray for the strength to find ways to comfort my mother in those moments of unknowing. I pray for strength to be unafraid of the future, especially when the moment comes in time when she will not remember me at all. I am strong thanks to my belief."

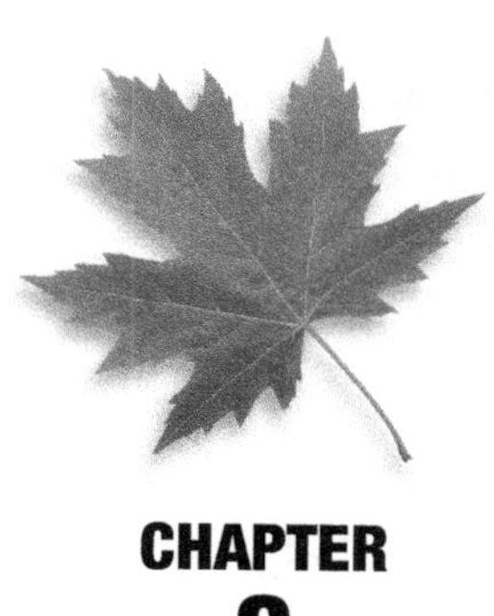

CHAPTER 8

The Power of Music With Dementia Residents

If upon hearing, "It's the story of a lovely lady ..." or "You are my Sunshine ..." you are instantly reminded of your childhood, you know the power of musical memory. Songs tell the stories of our lives. They remind us of a special day, a good time, a first love, and even a favorite car.

You maybe can't summon inspiration with a flick of the radio dial, or a tap on your iPod, but music can set the stage for creativity. Certain types of sounds can stimulate alpha waves in the elderly brain, which normally occur when you're close to sleep. The relaxed sensations created by alpha waves can lower the patients' mental barriers and help them to see new connections and possibilities.

Music therapy holds so many promises for many types of diseases; not only for memory loss, but also for working with people who have movement disorders, as well as behavior problems due to dementia/Alzheimer's disease.

Research has shown that music is one of our most persistent

memories and indeed can enhance and help in the recall of people, places, and events. Oliver Sacks, a neurologist and author of the book, *Musicophilia: Tales of Music and the Brain,* details how music is stored in the brain. His studies reveal that the music genres we learn and love in our teens and early 20s are the musical styles that will remain our favorites throughout our lives. These are the tunes that are most closely linked to our memories.

Any CD including *You are my Sunshine* is one of those albums that can bring so much joy to any long-term care community. It is rare to find CDs to which activity directors can conduct the whole morning stretch program, but they are out there.

Experiment with using music to spur your residents' creative juices by remembering these guidelines:

- **Don't play music nonstop.** It may distract them when they need to focus their attention on details. The best time is usually the mid-afternoon, to get through the post-lunch energy slump.
- **Choose the right music.** What is right? That depends on the residents' tastes, and current physical and/or mental conditions. Many researchers find that classical music of the baroque style relaxes minds and makes the patients more receptive to a unique activity program and care approach.
- **Be patient.** Just turning on a song will not instantly turn residents into fully alert and oriented individuals. Feed their minds in other ways, also; use art, games, and sufficient rest

so that they are ready and able to be creative when the time is right or during activity programs.

The power of the musical memory is so strong that for a brief moment a resident can leave their anxiety, confusion, and pain behind. This finding was confirmed by The National Institute of Nursing Research, where researchers found that music can reduce stress and pain levels. The National Institute of Education and Health Sciences reported music tempo can affect and improve mood and heart rate—a fact well known by everyone who has ever felt a bit down and turned on a radio to lighten their spirits!

Musical tastes and selections may be misunderstood among the generations, but the power of music crosses all age groups from The Rat Pack to the Fab Four, and ties notes to memories for a lifetime.

I have always known that music can open hearts. Through my personal experiences, I have seen how it can also open minds.

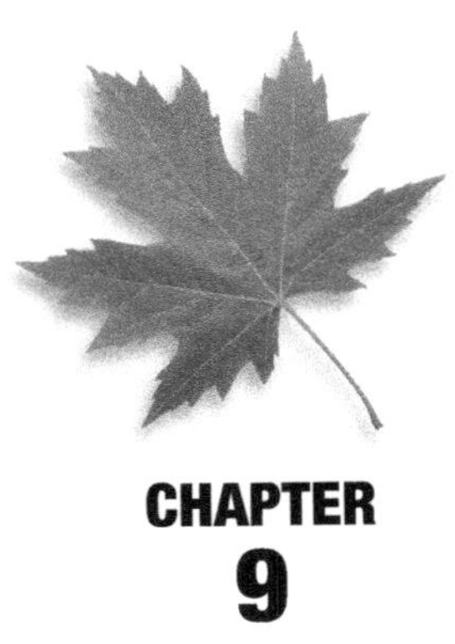

CHAPTER 9

Tips for Effective Communication With Memory-Impaired Loved Ones

Both family and paid caregivers may overlook various barriers to effective communication with impaired older adults and consequently misinterpret verbal and behavioral messages.

When someone has Alzheimer's disease, or any other form of memory impairment, communication can become more difficult. The patient's understanding of what you are saying and their ability to make you understand their world can be highly variable, and each person will react to different stimuli in different ways. This means that we have to be sensitive to the way we present ourselves and how we give information when we talk to someone with Alzheimer's or other forms of dementia.

For the most effective way to talk and communicate with someone who has Alzheimer's, it is important to remember a few simple rules:

1) Body language has an impact on communication.

Your facial expression, your body language, the tone of your voice, all become extra-important when talking and communicating with someone with neurological problems. If a person with dementia feels threatened, undermined, or confused by your communication with them, they may react in a negative way to your interventions: i.e., conversation or information you provide can increase agitation, undermine their confidence, and increase their feelings of isolation.

2) Environmental awareness aids communication.

Is the lighting sufficient to aid communication? In conversation we usually look at the face and body of the person talking to us. The visual cues help us to understand content and intent. Make sure you have some light on your face. Be aware of the limitations of communication in a dark room through the night.

3) Identify yourself and address the person by name.

This helps someone with Alzheimer's to orient themselves.

4) Does the person with dementia have hearing or sight difficulties?

Make allowances for visual and hearing deficits. Evaluate the potential of a medical evaluation to identify hearing/visual aids that can assist communication.

5) Be sure that you have the person's attention.

6) Speak slowly, calmly, and distinctly.

For effective communication you need to balance distinctive speech with not treating the person with dementia as you would a child, and without shouting or becoming angry with them if they do not understand. Shouting also affects the tone of your voice and makes understanding more difficult. Do not get angry even if you find yourself becoming frustrated. We all have seen people talking too loudly to people with dementia; it is unkind and it really does not help their self-respect and confidence.

7) Use simple, direct statements and information.

- Use words the person can understand.
- Do not give more than one instruction at a time.
- Do not press for an answer if the question worries or confuses them.
- Ask questions that require a "yes" or "no" response if that aids conversation and understanding.

8) Recognize that you may not understand the content of their conversation.

If you do not understand what they have said you can ask them to repeat it. Sometimes conversing with individuals with Alzheimer's is not necessarily about understanding; rather, it is about showing care, concern, inclusion, and love towards them.

9) Correcting wrong information.

It is not necessary to constantly correct the validity of the person's statement when it includes wrong information.

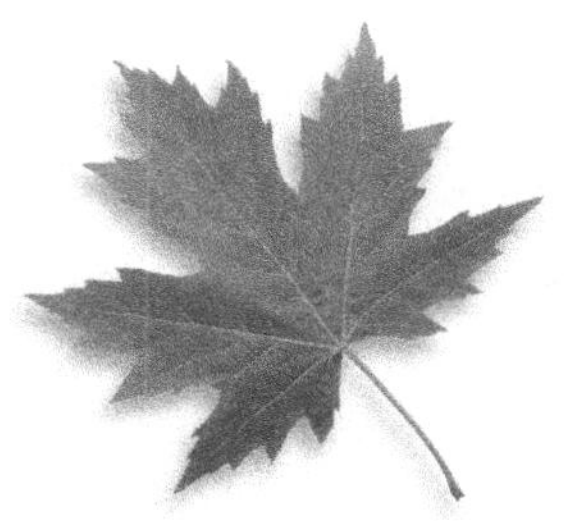

CHAPTER 10

Medication: Special Concerns in Dementia and Alzheimer's Patients

Many older adults must take several medications each day as they strive to keep their health in balance and remain independent. As many as 10 percent of people who are over age 65 take five or more prescription drugs, requiring them to juggle potentially dozens of pills every day. Painful arthritis may make opening a pill bottle seem as difficult as crushing a stone. Failing vision might prevent some older adults from reading key warning labels or instructions.

The Beers Criteria for Potentially Inappropriate Medication Use in Older Adults, commonly called the "Beers List," is a guideline first prepared by Dr. Mark Beers in 1991 for healthcare professionals, to help improve the safety of prescribing medications for older adults. The criteria are used in geriatrics clinical care to monitor and improve the quality of healthcare. The criteria are also used in clinical care, training, research, and healthcare policy to develop performance measures and document outcomes. The "Beers Criteria" contains lists of medications that pose potential risks outweighing potential benefits for people 65 and older. By considering this information during routine care, practitioners may prevent harmful side effects, including those that could be life-threatening or pose other "adverse drug events." As more people reach geriatric status, the delivery of safe and effective healthcare in this special population has become increasingly important.

While a medication organizer, pill bottle opener, or magnifying glass can help to overcome some of the medication-taking obstacles, we cannot prevent the normal aging process that causes side effects from medications. Both the liver's ability to inactivate drugs and the kidneys' ability to get rid of drugs slow with age. Beers warns that a doctor must lower the dosage of certain drugs to prevent over-medicating and to avoid causing side effects.

Several key factors place older adults at greater risk for reactions to medication, including falls, confusion or drowsiness, and medication-related hospital admissions. Both you and your doctor must work together to minimize potential medication-related pitfalls.

Tips for Medication Use by Older Adults

The more medications someone takes, the greater the risk for a drug reaction, particularly with increasing age. Furthermore, it is not unusual for doctors to prescribe the same dose of a medication for both a 200-pound athlete and a 90-pound older adult with chronic illnesses. Weight and size do matter. The volume of muscle (lean body) mass decreases with aging, as the body stores more fat cells. Body size, percent fat, and how lubed and primed the kidneys are can significantly affect dosing of popular drugs such as antibiotics (cephalosporins, penicillins, quinolones), heart drugs (digoxin, atenolol, ACE inhibitors), and even the household pain reliever acetaminophen. Taking medication comes down to a risk versus benefit analysis. Here are a few basic guidelines:

- Be certain that your doctor periodically reevaluates all medications the patient takes for possible dosage adjustments, drug-drug reactions, drug-disease side effects, and to determine if a drug can be safely discontinued.
- Anne L. Hume, Pharm. D., Professor and Chair of the Department of Pharmacy Practice at the University of Rhode Island, advises older adults to always ask if a drug can make them drowsy or dizzy and if there are ways to reduce those effects.
- Tell your patient's doctor about any over-the-counter medications the patient takes as well as herbal remedies. These may interact with prescription medications or have side effects.
- Each time you renew a prescription, be sure you receive the same generic product. Different formulations of a medication can actually contain up to 10 percent more or less of the active ingredient.
- When a new prescription is initiated, clarify with the doctor how long the medication will be taken by the patient and how it should be taken.
- Beers advises patients to use their pharmacist as a resource for reviewing all medications to check for interactions. This

strategy is particularly useful if your doctor seems rushed when going over your medications.

- Be prepared with the right tools for the job. Purchase a pill splitter for a dose of only half a pill, as long as your pharmacist says that the drug can be split. A large magnifying glass can be useful for reading directions or warnings in small print. Many inexpensive pill bottle openers can help those who have difficulty opening child safety caps. In fact, if you tell your pharmacist that you cannot open safety caps and you have no children in your household, the pharmacist will use a cap that opens with less effort.
- Consider buying one of many pill-dispensing gadgets to help develop a system for properly taking all medication. Check with your local pharmacy or search the Web for options.
- Consider signing up for one of many available Internet services that send medication-taking reminders. Reminders can be in the form of telephone calls, e-mails, or a beeper.

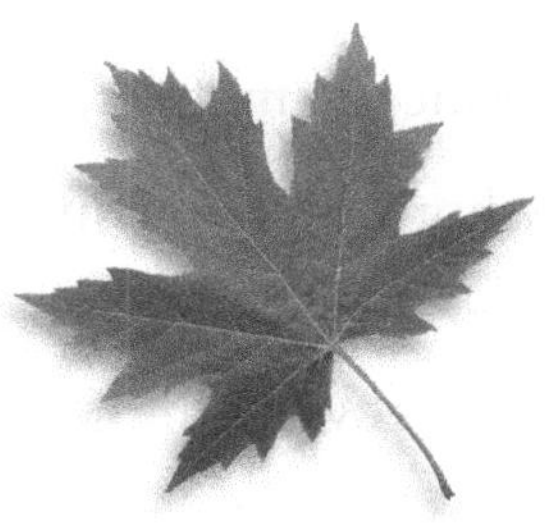

CHAPTER 11

Protect Your Memory-Impaired Loved Ones From Scammers

Adult children and caregivers play an important role in helping older people avoid scams. Oftentimes seniors are lonely and looking for someone to talk to, and unfortunately, scammers prey on this. Sit down and talk to your elderly parents or loved one. Remind them not to give out personal or financial information to a stranger, no matter how friendly or persistent the caller or visitor is. Even if someone claims to represent a well-known charity, your loved one should hang up the phone or close the door.

Here are some of the con artists' favorite senior-directed scams:

Telemarketing Fraud: fabulous offers. A scammer will call, send a letter, or e-mail alerting you that you have won a big prize or that you can buy a product, perhaps prescription drugs, at a great price.

Health Insurance Frauds and Fraudulent "Anti-Aging" Products.

- Never sign blank insurance claim forms.
- Never give blanket authorization to a medical provider to bill for services rendered.
- Ask your medical providers what they will charge and what you will be expected to pay out of pocket.
- Give your insurance/Medicare identification only to those who have provided you with medical services.

Counterfeit Prescription Drugs Fraud. Use caution when purchasing drugs on the Internet. Do not purchase medications from unlicensed online distributors or those who sell medications without a prescription. Reputable online pharmacies will have a seal of approval called the Verified Internet Pharmacy Practice Site (VIPPS), provided by the Association of Boards of Pharmacy in the United States.

Funeral and Cemetery Fraud. Be an informed consumer. Take time to call and shop around before making a purchase. Take a friend with you who may offer some perspective to help make difficult decisions. Funeral homes are required to provide detailed general price lists over the phone or in writing.

Reverse Mortgage Scams. Reverse mortgage scams are engineered by unscrupulous professionals in a multitude of real estate and financial services, and related entities to steal the equity from the property of unsuspecting senior citizens aged 62 or older. They also use these seniors to unwittingly aid the fraudsters in stealing equity from a flipped property.

Phony Mortgage Offers. If you have a bigger mortgage than you can afford comfortably, watch out for companies that offer to negotiate a payment plan or loan modification. The fraudster might claim to be affiliated with your lender. You might be told to pay up-front fees. If you're having trouble making your payments, call your lender or find a housing counselor approved by the U.S. Department of Housing and Urban Development (http://www.hud.gov/).

Phony Banks. Watch out for callers who claim to be from your bank or credit card company. They will tell you they have noticed suspicious activity on your credit card and want to check it with you. You will know the call is not legitimate if the caller asks for your credit card or Social Security number to confirm that he is talking to the right person.

Phony E-mails. Beware of e-mails from what purports to be a trusted institution asking for your Social Security number or account numbers. Phony Bank of America and Citibank messages are common. One prevalent scheme is an e-mail promising you a tax refund from the IRS—but the IRS doesn't send e-mails to taxpayers.

Investment Schemes. If you think you can tell a con artist from a legitimate adviser, consider this finding from a major study: investment-fraud victims are more financially literate than non-victims. The reason that even knowledgeable investors still become victims of investment schemes is the nature of the hook used by the con artists: a promise of high returns with little risk. Think Bernard Madoff before you hand your money away.

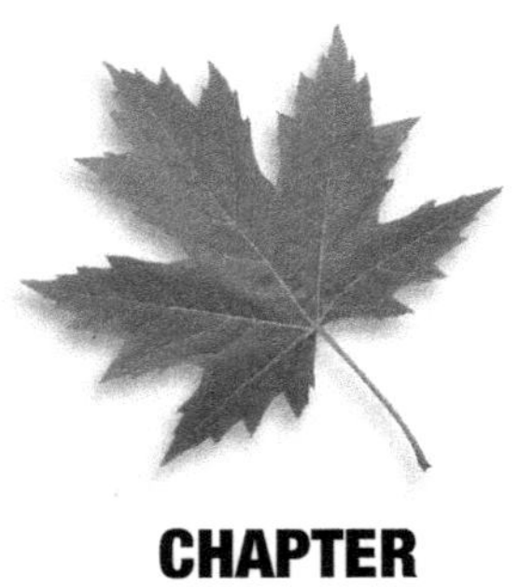

CHAPTER 12

Altering Caregiver Perceptions

At the root of all behavior is a purpose, although the cause may not be immediately known. Behavior is a response to the environment, to caregivers, or to internal stimuli. Problems may develop when the expectations of the caregiver do not match the abilities of the patient. The patient has a need for supervision and assistance because of increasing functional disability. The management of behavior is directed toward adapting the environment and approaches to the needs of the individual. Caregivers cannot cure the disease or teach patients to remember. They cannot resolve behavioral issues by using logic, by trying to reason with the person, or by coaxing or using flattery. Caregivers should have a healthy sense of humor and be flexible, creative, and patient.

The medical model of care is no longer effective for late-stage Alzheimer's disease (AD) patients. Rigid routines that require vital signs to be taken at 8 a.m., showers/baths to be completed by 11 a.m., and all residents in bed by 8 p.m. are unnecessary and unworkable. Creativity allows the caregiver to acknowledge that sleeping in a bed wearing nightclothes is not necessarily the "norm" for AD patients. Behavioral management is successful when caregivers can enter the patient's reality and utilize techniques that show respect for adult feelings rather than dwelling on childlike behavior. The behavior of a cognitively impaired person is logical within his or her own frame of reference. Knowledge of the patient's history is helpful to the caregiver, as it facilitates understanding the person who is reliving the 1930s, 1940s, or 1950s. An awareness of the patient's personal history is essential because it helps to know where the individual is "coming from" when he or she relives the past.

Avoid the use of labels in describing behavior. Words such as "uncooperative" are subjective and usually mean that the patient will not complete the desired task when asked to do so. When caregivers (hired or family) use such labels, the tone is set for all future contacts with the patient. Subsequent caregivers may thereafter assume from the label that the patient will be difficult, and thus actually elicit the poor behavior that is expected.

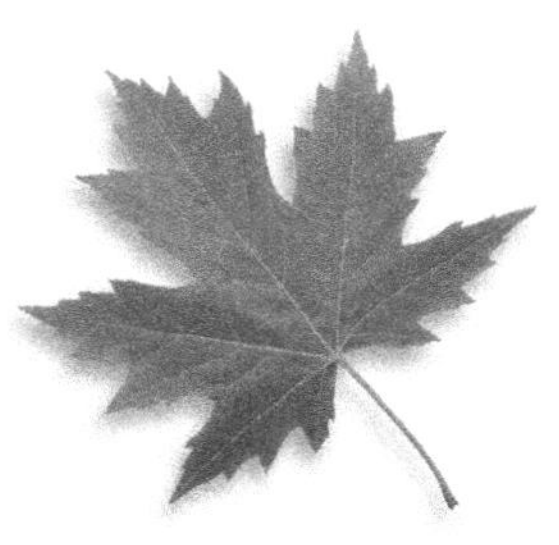

CHAPTER 13

Be a Happy, Enthusiastic Caregiver!

No one likes to work with a grouch.

When Norman Vincent Peale (author of *The Power of Positive Thinking*) said, "Be interesting, be enthusiastic ... and don't talk too much," he knew what he was talking about. He knew how you can brighten the day of the elder you care for. If you follow his advice, both you and your elders will benefit.

Here's why: your elders are like everyone else—they want to be near enthusiastic people who truly care and listen, who are energetic, and who are genuinely interested in their well-being.

You can find many published research projects demonstrating that caregiving with a smile and happy demeanor is effective; it can help improve your elder's depression and sadness. The problem is that many people feel unhappy much of the time, so it is difficult for them to appear happy during their caregiving work.

If you are one of those, here is something interesting for you to ponder: there have been recent reports showing that most of us can choose to be happy if we want to. We can learn how to be much happier each day, similarly to learning almost anything else.

Some tips on acquiring a happy attitude include:

- First, simply decide that you're going to be happy, each and every day. Make this decision early in the day, just as you are beginning your day. Try to avoid thinking negative thoughts. Many unhappy people think about negative things too much.
- If you can start thinking happy, positive thoughts, you will be a much happier person. Eventually, researchers tell us, thinking positive thoughts can become a regular habit, which helps to change your personality from worried to happy. Give it a try! Try being extra nice to people you see during the day. This can have a positive effect on you, too, and make you a happier person in addition to making your elders happier.
- Get involved in hobbies and social activities that you enjoy.

No one can be happy who constantly works and worries all the time. You need to do relaxing things that you enjoy. Once you have figured out how to be a happier, more enthusiastic person, you will want to take your new personality to your elders in ways that will make them happy, too.

Here is a suggestion on how you may be able to do this effectively: pretend you are an elder, and think about what would make you feel good, wanted, and cared for. For instance:

- You would understand that the caregiver has a private life, but would not want it to interfere with your care.
- You would also understand that your caregiver, whether a family member, an agency-hired caregiver, or part of the staff in a facility, may experience misunderstandings on occasion, but you would not want to hear about it or be a part of it.
- You would want your caregiver to know that you want to enjoy life, anticipate what could happen next, and have the chance to experience spontaneity and excitement.
- You would want to feel important to your caregivers and be their number one priority.

So, what are some ways to brighten the day of each of your elders?

Here are some suggestions for starters. You can probably think of many others. These suggestions are appropriate for the family member caring for a loved one at home, a paid caregiver helping in the home setting, or caregivers in a long-term facility. Create your own list and become the star caregiver who all family members and co-workers will envy day in and day out!

- Be yourself.
- Smile—always have a genuine smile on your face. Smile even if you don't feel like it ... because, after you smile, you *will* feel like it!
- Leave your personal worries and problems at home or share them with someone other than the loved one for whom you are caregiver; everyone has their own problems so do not share yours with your elders.

- Learn something new every day. You will feel good about it and will have something interesting to share.
- Be attentive; give your consideration and your time. Listen—don't talk too much. Give your elders the chance to talk and be heard. Learn when to be silent.
- Encourage conversation, even if answers are in the form of head nods.
- Do random acts of kindness; anticipate needs and "get there first." Participate in unplanned moments; for example, display the spontaneous side of you through song, dance, and hugs. Elders also love to be spontaneous.
- Make each elder feel special each day. Accept each of them "as is" and work with individual habits and traits.
- Look for special qualities in each and help each of them to grow.

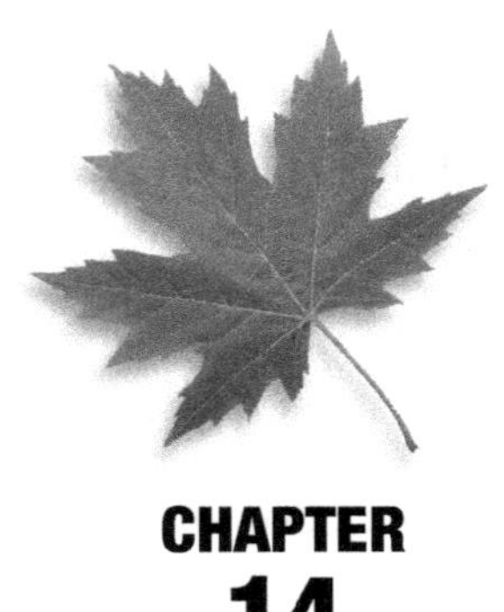

CHAPTER 14

Common Myths of Aging

The term "ageism" was coined by Robert Butler, M.D., in 1968. Dr. Butler is a geriatrician who saw that society had developed myths, stereotypes, and misunderstandings about people as they age. Like "racism" and "sexism," people who express ageism make general statements that are not true. Terms such as these imply that one group is inherently superior to another. We quickly see that denying a man a job because of his color is "racist" and believing that women should never work outside the home is "sexist." Ageism makes judgments about the actions, character, and desires of people based on their age. There is also a sense that old age is inferior to youth.

Ageism has developed over many years, as our society as a whole began to put a greater value on youth than on aging. Television, movies, and the printed media tend to strengthen the idea that young is "good" and old is "bad."

People who have little or no contact with elderly people are more likely to accept the myths and stereotypes of aging. People may visit their grandparents or see other elderly people while shopping, but many people never spend any time getting to know an elderly person as an individual. Those young people who believe the stereotypes see no reason to become close to an old person, as they perceive that elders have little to offer.

People may also believe the myths of aging because information about normal aging is scarce. As the size of the elderly population has grown, interest in research on aging has increased. Early research was found to be invalid due to the subjects chosen, so until recently, reliable information about the aging process has not been available.

Society holds several myths about the elderly. Many of these myths may be easily disputed based on data from the U.S. Census and other studies.

Myth: Dementia is an inevitable part of aging.

Fact: Dementia should be seen as a modifiable health condition and, if it occurs, should be followed as a medical condition, not a normal part of aging. In other words, if you or your loved one becomes forgetful, it could be related to medication, nutrition, or modifiable medical issues. Don't assume it is Alzheimer's.

Just consider that when doctors examined the brain of a 115-year-old woman, who at the time of her death was the world's oldest woman, they found essentially normal brain tissue, with no evidence of Alzheimer's or other dementia-causing conditions. Testing in the years before she died showed no loss in brain function.

Not only is dementia not an inevitability of aging, but you actually have some control over whether or not you develop it. Studies find that many of the same risk factors that contribute to heart disease—high blood pressure, high cholesterol, diabetes, and obesity—may also contribute to Alzheimer's and other dementias (http://www.healthywomen.org/glossary/term/5000). For instance, studies on the brains of elderly people with and without dementia find significant blood vessel damage in those with hypertension. Such damage shrinks the amount of healthy brain tissue you have in reserve, reducing the amount available if a disease such as Alzheimer's develops. That is important, because we are starting to understand that the more brain function you initially possess, the more you can afford to lose before your core functions are affected.

One way to dodge the dementia bullet is to exercise your body and your brain. Physical activity plays a role in reducing the risk of diseases that contribute to eventual Alzheimer's. It also builds up that brain reserve. One study, published in 2011, found that just one year of added regular physical activity contributed to increased brain volume in 60 otherwise healthy, but previously couch-potato individuals, aged 55 to 80 (Erickson et al., *PNAS* 2001, 108[7]:3017). A Tufts University research study performed during the 1980s and 90s finds that people who exercised twice a week over an average of 21 years slashed their risk of Alzheimer's in half.

Then there is intellectual exercise. It doesn't matter what kind of mental challenge you accept, only that you break out of your comfort zone. Even writing letters twice a week instead of sending e-mails can have brain-strengthening benefits. That is because such novel activities stimulate more regions of the brain, increasing blood flow and helping to not only build brain connections, but also to improve the health of existing tissue.

Myth: Life satisfaction is low among the elderly.

Fact: In 1991, Field and Millsap published in the *Journal of Gerontology*, an analysis of data from the Berkeley Older Generation Study which found that many elders are quite satisfied with their lives. More than one-third (36 percent) of persons older than 59 years of age, and 15 percent of those older than 79 years of age, stated that they were currently experiencing the best time in their lives.

The Berkeley Older Generation Study is unique and extremely informative, spanning 60 years of longitudinal investigation of the various developmental stages of life. Parents of children born in Berkeley, California, were randomly selected for inclusion in the study. The parents were interviewed as young adults, middle-aged adults, young-old adults (ages 65-75), and old-old adults (over 85). Field examined the responses given by participants as young-old adults and old-old adults. The two specific interview questions that tapped into happiness with life were: 1) "Looking back, what period of your life brought you the most satisfaction?" and 2) "What period brought you the least satisfaction?" In responding to the first question, the largest percentage of young-old interviewees selected the decade of their 50s as the most satisfying. When this same question was posed to the interviewees 14 years later, the decades of the 20s, 30s, 40s, and 60s were selected with nearly equal frequency as the most satisfying life period. When questioned about the least satisfying life period, interviewees who were young-old and old-

old selected their childhood and adolescence periods. Contrary to the myth of the youth-obsessed older adult, the era of childhood does not become more cherished with age.

Myth: Old people feel old.

Fact: According to a 2009 telephone survey conducted by the AARP, only 21 percent of individuals 65 to 74 years of age stated they felt old, and only 35 percent of those 75 years of age and older reported feeling old.

Myth: Old people are sexless.

Fact: There is a strong belief in our society that sex is for the young and that older people should not and/or cannot engage in sexual activity. Old and young people believe this myth. Many older people stop sexual relations because they have learned it is "bad" for them to continue. Elderly people who continue to have sex often feel guilty. Either way, it has a devastating emotional effect on them.

Research has found that sexual activity and enjoyment do not decrease with age. People with physical health, a sense of well-being, and a willing partner are more likely to continue sexual relations. People who are bored with their partner, mentally or physically tired, afraid of failure, or who overindulge in food or drink are unlikely to engage in sexual activity. These reasons do not differ a great deal when considering whether or not a person will engage in sex at any age.

Myth: Old people are inflexible.

Fact: Inflexibility means to be resistant to change and to be unable to adapt to new situations. People of any age can be inflexible. Increased age does not make a person inflexible, and in fact, the opposite is true. Older people must adjust to changes such as retirement, disease, illness, death of family and/or friends, and lifestyle. Without the ability to accept change, adjustment to these changes would be impossible. Research shows that older people may change their opinion more slowly than younger people, but most remain open to change throughout their lives.

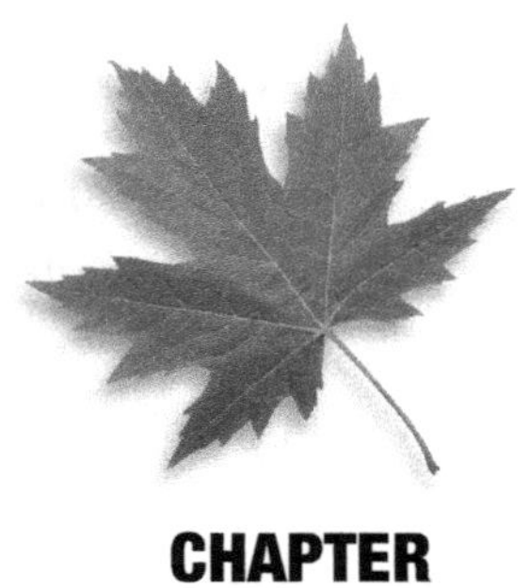

CHAPTER 15

Defining and Understanding Culture Change

A growing number of care providers and elder advocates are taking dramatic steps to revise longstanding negative stereotypes of the long-term care home by creating both home and community environments that appeal to elders, employees, and visitors alike. The transformation that these facilities and care providers are undertaking amounts to a virtual cultural shift, known in the industry as culture change.

Culture change is receiving growing popularity in the senior living industry; however, the majority of organizations have yet to begin tackling this transformation. One of the contributions to this hesitancy may be that no universal explicit definition of culture change is accepted within the industry.

This new approach to treating the elderly involves redefining and recreating long-term care by altering the organizational culture, the operations, and the physical setting away from traditional medical/institutional approaches and toward a humanistic approach. Culture change requires a new attitude and a sense of purpose, both of which may conflict with old-style caregiving routines. This type of transformation is complex, time-consuming, and often personally challenging for those involved.

Although discovering a definition of culture change in long-term care will not remove all the challenges and struggles faced by those who take on this transformation, a succinct definition of culture change in long-term care may assist in setting goals, planning changes, and understanding this transformative process.

The three most important segments of culture change that I am a true advocate for are:

- removing the institutional medical model of long-term care;
- humanizing the facility by valuing individuals and their rights, freedoms, and/or capabilities; and
- becoming resident-focused through utilizing a person-centered care model.

Person-centered care is defined as the philosophical foundation of gerontological nursing. This policy requires an active relationship between healthcare professionals and elder individuals who require assistance in order to "provide that assistance in such a way that clients are honored and valued and are not lost in the tasks of caregiving" (Crandall et al., *Journal of Gerontological Nursing* 2007, 33([11]:47).

While some worry that a resident-centered care approach will make life harder for long-term care home staff while de-emphasizing the quality of clinical care provided, the evidence so far suggests the opposite. Yet, as the movement has gained momentum, it has become clear that resident-centered care needs to be measurable. Long-term care facilities must be able to identify the steps required and to assess their progress along the way.

There are five areas within an organization that are transformed by culture change:

- decision-making,
- leadership,
- staff roles,
- the physical environment,
- and organizational design.

In the culture change model, greater control is given to "frontline" workers—the nurse aides who handle so much of the day-to-day care of residents—as well as family members and residents. Additionally, staff members are permanently assigned to a particular group of residents as members of self-directed work teams. Rather than working in a single department, such as nursing, housekeeping, or food service, staff functions are blended so that all staff members can help residents with their personal care, lead activities, and do cooking and light housekeeping.

Experience has demonstrated that if change in the culture of dementia care is to occur in long-term care facilities, a catalyst for change or a change agent must step forward to identify the new vision of care and to take responsibility on a continuing basis for the process of culture change in their facilities (Fagan, Williams, and Burger, 1997 [presentation]; Coons, D.H., 1992 [personal communication]; Peppard, N., 1991, Springer Publishing Co.; Hiatt, Merlino, and Ronch, 1987 [Conference Proceedings, Albany, New York State Department of Health]). The change agent must be a leader, i.e., a person with interpersonal and intellectual resources, respected by co-workers, and who can inspire confidence and convey a sense of security in a changing workplace. The literature has identified a constellation of attributes and capabilities that are regarded as most desirable in a culture change agent.

The attributes include:

- Ability to lead without being controlling;
- Skilled at giving support and facilitating interaction;
- Open to the ideas of others;
- Able to assume full responsibility for his or her actions;
- Willing and able to share knowledge;
- Able to establish clear criteria for good job performance.

The agents can:

- Assist staff to achieve personal work-related development;
- Convey the philosophy that this work is "rewarding";
- Help staff recognize both individual and team success;
- Help staff go beyond their job description to give quality care;
- Avoid being discouraged by failure, but rather learn from it;

- Communicate comfort with, and excitement about, trying new ideas;
- Delegate responsibility, not just work;
- Engage people's unique personal gifts in addition to their professional abilities;
- Treat team members as valued equals.

The agents have:

- An abundance of creative energy;
- A clear grasp of the new culture of dementia care and can communicate why it is important;
- Knowledge about long-term care administration;
- Administrative and management experience;
- The drive to continue gerontological or geriatric training.

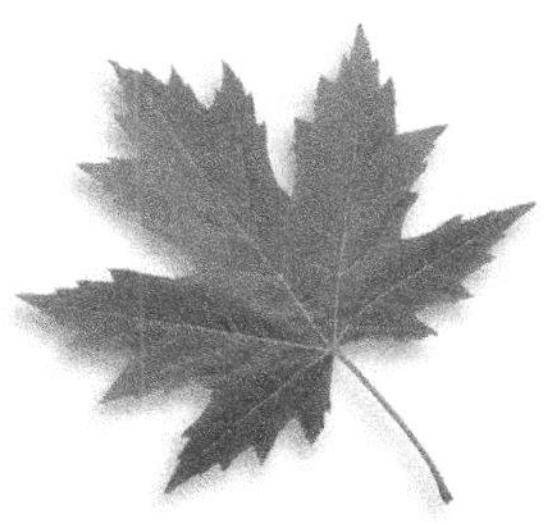

CHAPTER 16

Abuse and Neglect of the Alzheimer's Patient—Red Flags

Elder Abuse is one of the most overlooked public health hazards in the United States. The National Center on Elder Abuse estimates that between one and two million elderly adults have suffered from some form of elder abuse. The primary types of elder abuse are physical abuse, sexual abuse, emotional and psychological abuse, neglect and self-neglect, abandonment, and financial exploitation. Elders with dementia are thought to be at greater risk of abuse and neglect than those of the general elderly population.

One occasionally reads sensationalized newspaper stories of elderly Alzheimer's and dementia victims who were subjected to abuse or neglect while they were residents in a long-term care facility. Based on such newspaper accounts, one would have the impression that most cases of the abuse or neglect of Alzheimer's or dementia victims take place in such facilities. While such sorry events and incidents do take place in long-term care facilities, they are rare and far from the norm. Recent studies, however, have established rather clearly, the troubling fact that most cases of the abuse of Alzheimer's and dementia victims actually take place in the family home setting, by their own family members, or paid caregivers.

Potential Indicators of Abuse

Below are some potential indicators for each type of elder abuse. Please be aware that this does not represent a definitive listing.

Passive and active neglect

- Evidence that personal care is lacking or neglected
- Signs of malnourishment (e.g., sunken eyes, loss of weight)
- Chronic health problems, both physical and/or psychiatric
- Dehydration (extreme thirst)
- Pressure sores (bed sores)

Physical Abuse

- Overt signs of physical trauma (e.g., scratches, bruises, cuts, burns, punctures, choke marks)
- Signs of restraint trauma injury, particularly if repeated (e.g., sprains, fractures, detached retina, dislocation, paralysis)
- Additional physical indicators, such as hypothermia, abnormal chemistry values, pain upon being touched
- Repeated "unexplained" injuries
- Inconsistent explanations of the injuries

- A physical examination revealing that the older person has injuries which the caregiver has failed to disclose
- A history of doctor or emergency room "shopping"
- Repeated time lags between the time of any "injury or fall" and medical treatment

Material or Financial Abuse

- Unusual banking activity, or bank statements (credit card statements, etc.) no longer being sent directly to the elder adult
- Documents are being drawn up for the elder to sign but the elder cannot explain or understand the purpose of the papers
- The elder's living situation is not commensurate with the size of the elder's estate (e.g., lack of new clothing or amenities, unpaid bills)
- The caregiver only expresses concern regarding the financial status of the elder person and does not ask questions or express concern regarding the physical and/or mental health status of the elder
- Personal belongings such as jewelry, art, furs are missing
- Signatures on checks and other documents do not match the signature of the elder
- Recent acquaintances, housekeepers, "care" providers, etc., declare undying affection for the older person and isolate the elder from long-term friends or family
- Recent acquaintances, housekeepers, caregivers, etc., make promises of lifelong care in exchange for deeding all

property and/or assigning all assets over to the acquaintance, caregiver, etc.

Psychological Abuse

- Psychological Signs:

  Ambivalence, deference, passivity, shame

  Anxiety (mild to severe)

  Depression, hopelessness, helplessness, thoughts of suicide

  Confusion, disorientation

- Behavioral Signs:

  Trembling, clinging, cowering, lack of eye contact

  Evasiveness

  Agitation

  Hypervigilance

Sexual Abuse

- Trauma to the genital area (e.g., bruises)
- Venereal disease
- Infections/unusual discharge or smell
- Indicators common to psychological abuse may be concomitant with sexual abuse

Violation of basic rights

- Caregiver withholds or reads the elder's mail
- Caregiver intentionally obstructs the elder person's religious observances (e.g., dietary restrictions, holiday

participation, visits by minister/priest/rabbi, etc.)

- Caregiver has removed all doors from the elder adult's rooms
- As violation of basic rights is often concomitant with psychological abuse, the indicators of basic rights violations are similar indicators as those for psychological abuse

Self-Neglect

This is a controversial category in relation to elder abuse. The following questions lie at the heart of the controversy: 1) If an individual is competent but chooses to neglect their personal health or safety, is this abuse? 2) Is intervention, particularly unsolicited intervention, appropriate in cases of self-neglect?

Self-neglect, if included statistically as a form of elder abuse, represents the highest percentage of cases of elder abuse. In fact, the Public Policy Institute of AARP estimates that self-neglect represents 40 to 50 percent of cases reported to states' Adult Protective Services.

Unfortunately, these statistics fail to take into account the fact that self-abusers do not fit a uniform profile. There are many factors which may lead one to self-neglect and the subsequent intervention necessary for each is unique.

Family Abuse

Although many family caregivers gain satisfaction from their role, there are negative aspects to caring for a dementia-impaired person. Caregivers of people with dementia often experience greater strain and distress than caregivers of other elder people. Caring for a family member with dementia can be a life-changing and very demanding experience. Often people who start caring for a family member do not feel adequately prepared for the role.

As people with dementia try to deal with their experience of dementia, they may sometimes exhibit behavior that seems aggressive or violent. This behavior can be highly stressful for caregivers (https://www.alzheimers.org.uk/site/scripts/documents.php?categoryID=200343) and is highly predictive of mistreatment and abuse on the part of the caregivers. There is considerable evidence that caregiver and care-worker stress impacts the level of support they can provide; therefore, greater understanding about dementia and ways of working with people with dementia can reduce caregivers' stress and improve their ability to provide positive support.

Family abuse can be considered from two perspectives: abuse that is perpetrated deliberately, and abuse that is not. Sometimes the level of care and support is inadequate because the perpetrator is not capable of providing it even while doing his or her best. Sometimes it is because they aren't aware of the care and support services available to them, and sometimes the reason is that the necessary support is not available. Abuse which is not deliberate can include a wide range of actions, including neglect or unnecessary restraint of a person with dementia.

Regardless of whether or not the abuse is perpetrated deliberately, from the perspective of the victim the impact is the same. For this reason, all forms of abuse are unacceptable and equally subject to the law.

It is also important to note that people with dementia can themselves abuse their caregivers. This is usually due to the behavioral and psychological symptoms of dementia, which may include depression, loss of inhibitions, and aggression.

There is widespread failure to supply an adequate number and choice of services for people with dementia and their caregivers. Support services for caregivers can be an essential source of emotional and practical support, and can empower the caregivers to care for the person with dementia. In particular, these services can include:

- Training in the best ways of caring for a person with dementia, and education about the symptoms of dementia, particularly behavioral and psychological symptoms;
- Peer support networks such as *Talking Point* (http://www.alzheimers.org.uk/site/scripts/documents_info.php?documentID=1077);
- Access to flexible and good-quality short breaks;
- Psychological support;
- Information about rights and entitlements.

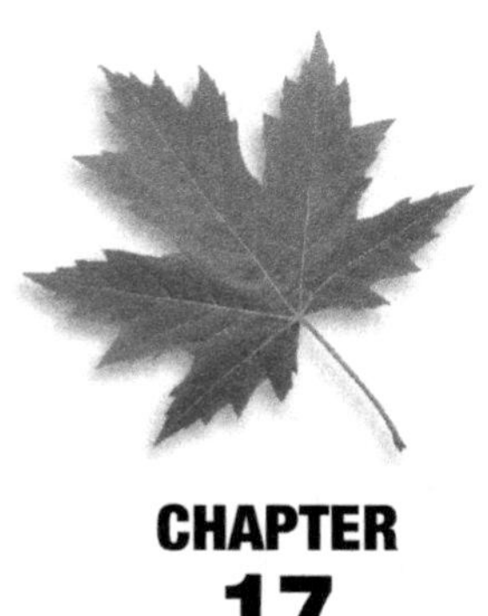

CHAPTER 17

HIPAA: Questions and Answers for Family Caregivers

Suppose your mother is a patient in the hospital or emergency room. You are her family caregiver and when you ask about her treatment, the doctor or nurse says, "I can't tell you that because of HIPAA."

That answer is incorrect. But you need to know more. What is HIPAA? Why should you, as a family caregiver, need to know your mother's medical information? And what can you do to get the information you need? Here are answers to these and other questions family caregivers ask about HIPAA.

What Is HIPAA?

HIPAA (Health Insurance Portability and Accountability Act) is a federal law that protects personal medical information. The law allows only certain people to see this information. This means that employers or groups who want this information for their own use cannot have it.

Who Are Family Caregivers?

A family caregiver is someone who takes care of a person who has a chronic or serious illness or disability. The caregiver can be a family member, friend, partner, or someone else close to the patient. He or she does not need to live with the patient.

Doctors and other health care professionals can share medical information with family caregivers or others directly involved with a patient's care. The only time this cannot happen is when the patient says he or she does not want this information shared with others.

Why Do Family Caregivers Need Medical Information?

Family caregivers need medical information so that they can better manage and provide care for the loved one. For example, they need to know what medical problem the person is being treated for. They need to know the names of the medicines the doctor orders, why the doctor thinks the patient needs them, and what side effects to monitor for.

Who Is Allowed to See a Patient's Medical Information?

Doctors and other health care professionals can share medical information with family caregivers or others directly involved with a patient's care. The only time this cannot happen is when the patient says he or she does not want this information shared with others. Sometimes there is more than one family caregiver. If so, it is a good idea to choose only one person to talk with the patient's doctor or medical team. This person can then share important information with health care professionals or other family caregivers who provide care. Doctors also share medical information with nurses, therapists, and other health care professionals on the patient's medical team. This is important for good care and is not affected by HIPAA.

Does the Patient Have to Sign Any Papers?

Some hospitals or other healthcare facilities ask patients to sign written consent forms before doctors discuss medical information with family caregivers. This is not part of the HIPAA law, but may be part of the healthcare facility's procedures.

What if I Have a Problem Getting Medical Information?

Talk with the social worker, patient representative, or privacy officer if you are the family caregiver and have trouble getting your patient's medical information. The next time your family member is a patient in the hospital or emergency room, tell the doctor or nurse that you are the person's family caregiver. The best care happens when the doctor or nurse then says, "Let's talk about the treatment your family member needs and how we can all help."

Ways to Learn More About HIPAA.

More information is available from the Department of Health and Human Services' Office for Civil Rights website at www.hhs.gov/ocr/hipaa and the_Health Privacy Project website at www.healthprivacy.org.

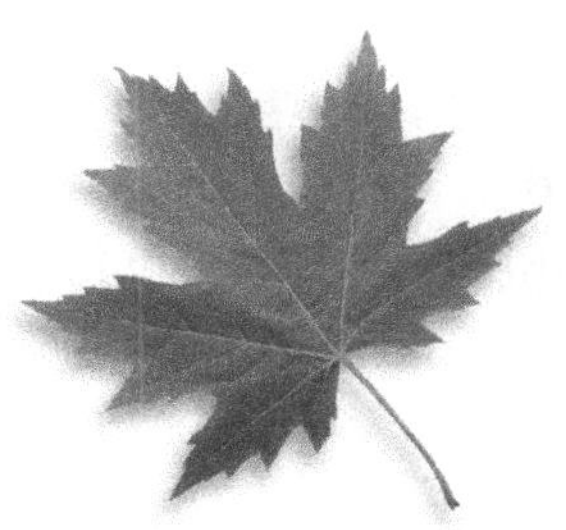

CHAPTER 18

How Hospital Observation Versus Admission Affects Alzheimer's Patients' Medicare Status

Hospitals have the ability to classify Medicare patients as an "observation" admission during the patient's stay. "Observation" admissions are apparently paid at a lower rate, but don't come under as much Medicare scrutiny. Additionally, under Medicare rules, "observation" patients may have to pay a 20 percent co-payment that wouldn't be required if they were admitted. Medicare "observation" patients also have to pay full price for any subsequent care that is rendered after they have been discharged.

Also note how Medicare is planning to penalize hospitals that re-admit too many patients, which will only increase the number of patients classified as "observation" status.

What are Observation Services?

Observation services are defined in Medicare's manuals as:

A well-defined set of specific, clinically appropriate services, which include ongoing short-term treatment, assessment, and reassessment, that are furnished while a decision is being made regarding whether patients will require further treatment as hospital inpatients or if they are able to be discharged from the hospital.

The manuals suggest that a patient may not remain in observation status for more than 24 hours. Since 2004, The Centers for Medicare and Medicaid Services (CMS) has authorized hospitalization utilization review (UR) committees to change a patient's status from inpatient to outpatient, retroactively, if (1) the change is made while the patient is still hospitalized; (2) the hospital has not submitted a claim to Medicare for the inpatient admission; (3) a physician concurs in the UR committee's decision; and (4) the physician's concurrence is documented in the patient's medical record (http://www.medicareadvocacy.org/observation-services-what-can-beneficiaries-and-advocates-do/). CMS anticipated that retroactive reclassifications would occur infrequently, "such as a late-night weekend admission when no case manager is on duty to offer guidance."

On one hand, hospitals get paid more for admitting Medicare patients. On the other, hospitals could be accused of false claims and penalized for admitting Medicare patients who don't meet Medicare's strict admission criteria. Medicare's Recovery Audit Contractors (RAC) will be combing through charts because they have a financial incentive to find patients who have been "inappropriately" classified as "admissions."

So hospitals play it safe and classify more and more Medicare patients as "observation" status.

Who gets stuck in the middle? It is the patients, many of whom worked their entire lives and paid into a system so that they would have medical care when they reached age 65.

What Should Beneficiaries and Their Advocates Do?

The Center for Medicare Advocacy suggests that beneficiaries file an appeal from any hospital notices describing their observation status and any subsequent Advanced Beneficiary Notice/Notice of Exclusion from Medicare Benefits they receive from a Skilled Nursing Facility (SNF, also known as a nursing home or rehab facility). In the likely absence of any notice, particularly from a hospital, the Center recommends that beneficiaries appeal when they receive the Medicare Summary Notice, which sets out all healthcare services received by a beneficiary in the prior quarter.

In all cases, beneficiaries and their advocates should gather the complete medical records from the hospital to establish the entire set of services and treatments that were received during the period of hospitalization. Advocates should request copies of all documents used by the hospital, its UR Committee, and outside consultants engaged by the hospital to determine the status of beneficiaries. Advocates should present the medical and nursing facts and cite any physician support for inpatient status to demonstrate that the beneficiary met Medicare's criteria for an inpatient stay. If SNF coverage is also an issue, advocates must demonstrate not only that the beneficiary met the criteria for Medicare-covered care in the SNF but also that the beneficiary *received* Medicare-covered care in the SNF.

Advocates should not be discouraged if they lose at the early stages of appeal. If you asked a Quality Improvement Organization (QIO) to review the hospital's decision to discharge you or your loved one, and the QIO decided against you, you can appeal that decision.

If the QIO decides against you and you (or the one for whom you are providing care) are still in the hospital, you can ask another organization, the Qualified Independent Contractor (QIC), for an immediate (expedited) reconsideration. To get one, you must call or write to the QIC by noon the day after you received the QIO's decision.

The QIC must immediately notify the hospital and QIO of the reconsideration request and allow you and the hospital to submit information. The QIC must notify you in writing of its decision within 72 hours of receipt of your request for an expedited determination, though the request must be accompanied by all necessary information to decide the case (you can request that this deadline be extended by up to 14 days if you need time to gather additional evidence; for example, if you need to get in touch with your doctor and he or she is out of town). The hospital cannot charge you for care until the QIC reaches its decision.

If the QIC misses the 72-hour deadline for reaching a decision, and you have not requested an extension, and at least $140 is at stake (in 2013), you can ask that the appeal be automatically transferred to the Administrative Law Judge (ALJ), the next level of appeal.

If you missed the deadline for the expedited reconsideration or you have left the hospital, you can request a standard reconsideration by the QIC within 180 days of receipt of the QIO's decision. The QIC generally has 60 days from your request for a reconsideration to notify you in writing of its decision or of your right to automatically transfer your case to the ALJ if at least $140 is at stake (in 2013).

The hospital can bill you before the QIC makes its decision, but must reimburse you any amounts you paid if the QIC later rules in your favor.

If the QIC decides against you, you can appeal its decision to the Administrative Law Judge.

Another point of concern for many patients should be Obama Care, or as it is known, the Affordable Care Act. Under new Obama Care rules, hospitals will have an incentive to "game" the system to improve their Medicare statistics, even at patient expense, by classifying more emergency room visits as "observation."

The Obama administration's latest focus for healthcare cost control is Medicare hospital readmissions. Nearly 20 percent of Medicare patients discharged from a hospital require re-hospitalization within 30 days, costing the government $17 billion per year. The federal government regards many of these readmissions as "avoidable," wasteful spending. Under Obama Care, the government has begun imposing financial penalties on hospitals deemed to be readmitting too many Medicare patients within 30 days for pneumonia, heart failure, or myocardial infarct (heart attack). The presumption is that the hospitals didn't provide proper care initially or didn't assure appropriate post-hospital care.

Recently, the federal government announced the first round of penalties. To many experts' surprise, the list included some of the nation's top hospitals: Massachusetts General Hospital (ranked #1 in the latest *US News* report), Barnes-Jewish Hospital in St. Louis, and University of Michigan Hospital. Over 2200 hospitals across the country were penalized.

In response, hospitals will undoubtedly seek to improve any truly substandard patient care. But many hospitals may also be tempted to game the system to improve their readmission statistics.

There is already worrisome precedent for such gaming. There is a sharp rise in the practice of hospitals transferring sick ER patients to short-term "observation" beds (for up to 72 hours sometimes), which don't count as true hospital admissions. This rise coincided with Medicare payment rules aimed at reducing hospital admissions. Hospital admissions fell, but patients received lower levels of care and likely incurred greater out-of-pocket expenses.

The Obama Care rules may also pressure doctors to delay readmissions. New doctors are increasingly choosing to become hospital employees rather than enter private practice. They could face significant conflicts of interest when they consider a patient readmission medically necessary but the hospital administrator thinks otherwise. Will doctors compromise patient care when their readmission statistics are being monitored by someone who can terminate their employment contract?

The Obama Care rules may lead to the perverse punishment of good hospitals. Several hospitals with above-average readmission rates also have below-average mortality rates. These include well-known centers such as Beth Israel Deaconess in Boston and Maimonides Medical Center in Brooklyn, New York. These hospitals have low mortality rates because they keep their sickest patients alive rather than letting them die. But those are patients who also are most likely to require future hospitalizations. Hence, these hospitals are being punished for doing a good job.

A recent *New England Journal of Medicine* article raised other serious concerns about the Obama Care policy (Joynt and Jha, 2012, *N Engl J Med*, 366:1366). The authors note that 30-day readmissions are often caused by factors outside a hospital's control, such as patient noncompliance with new medications or diet. Hospitals, in such cases, will "expend substantial energy yet have little effect." Furthermore, the penalties "will disproportionately affect institutions that care for poor or minority populations."

Although the Obama Care readmission rules initially apply only to Medicare patients, private insurers tend to follow Medicare payment guidelines. Thus, millions of Americans with private insurance could soon be affected as well.

The fundamental problem with the Obama administration's approach is that it forces hospitals and doctors to place the government's priorities ahead of their patients' needs. It is similar to government rewarding or punishing schools based on student performance on mandatory standardized tests. Schools inevitably end up "teaching for the test," rather than teaching students what is appropriate for future academic and life success.

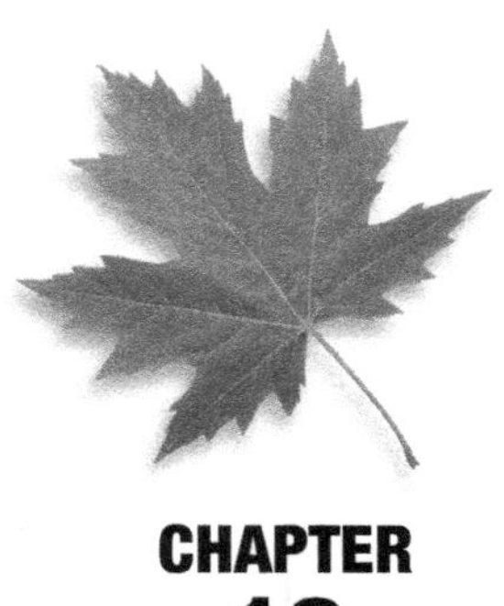

CHAPTER 19

The Alzheimer's Disease Patient Bill of Rights

Every person diagnosed with Alzheimer's disease or other dementia deserves:

- To be informed of one's diagnosis;
- To have appropriate, ongoing medical care;
- To be treated as an adult, listened to, and afforded respect for one's feelings and point of view;
- To be with individuals who know one's life story, including cultural and spiritual traditions;
- To experience meaningful engagement throughout the day;
- To live in a safe and stimulating environment;
- To be outdoors on a regular basis;
- To be free from psychotropic medications whenever possible;

- To receive welcomed physical contact, including hugging, caressing, and handholding;
- To be an advocate for oneself and for others;
- To be part of a local, global, or online community;
- To have care partners well trained in dementia care.

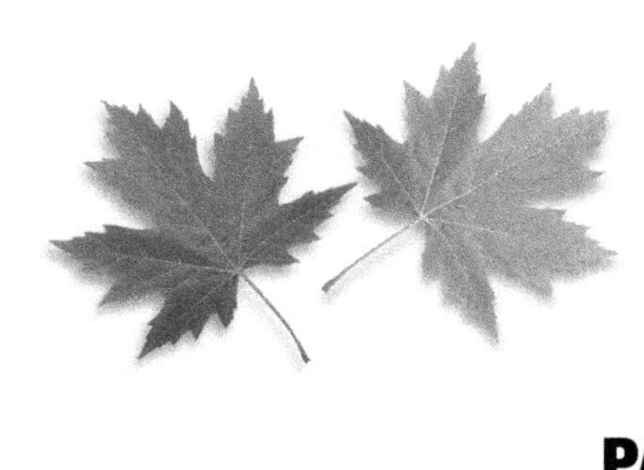

PART II
Care at Home

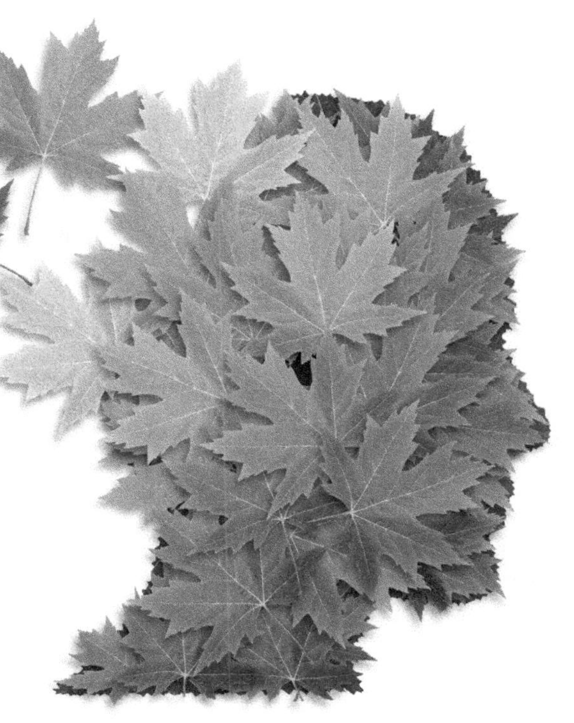

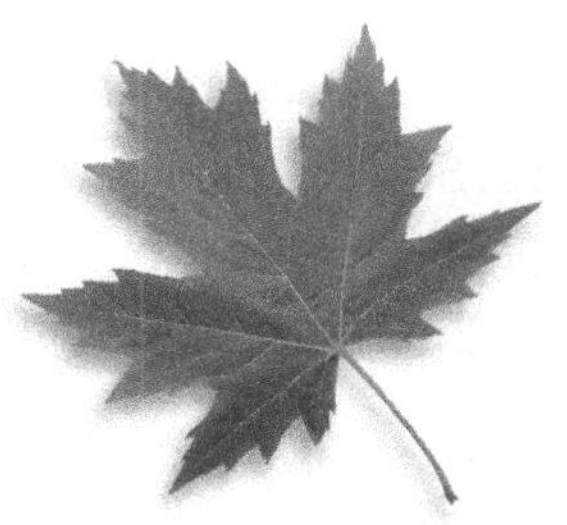

CHAPTER 20

Keeping Our Parents a Little Longer at Home and Providing a Safe Environment

It is a given that most elderly people want to stay in their homes and not in a long-term care facility. We as the family/caregivers need to assess the risks and the wishes of our parents. It is our responsibility to ensure their safety while they stay at home.

Physical Safety

- **Bathrooms:** Check the house for fall risks, stairs, grab-bars in the shower/tub. It is very important to secure the bathrooms since most falls happen after the shower. Secure the toilet with grab-bars and elevate the toilet seat. Replace all throw rugs in the bathroom and kitchen with nonskid rugs and place nonskid mats in the shower/tub.
- **Kitchen:** If our parents suffer from any memory impairment, we need to secure the kitchen. For instance, remove the aluminum foil from the kitchen, as they may warm their

meal in the microwave with aluminum foil covering the dish, creating a fire hazard. Secure all sharp objects. Using an automatic stove timer is great; and if possible, remove the oven knobs to prevent accidental natural gas hazards.

- **Medical Alarm System and Communication:** There are many available systems that provide elders the opportunity to call for help for any reason. Provide a phone that has large digits and is simple to work. Write the most important telephone numbers next to the phone on a board, as paper notes have a tendency to disappear. An amplified speaker phone will improve a phone conversation for those who have difficulty hearing.
- **Improve lighting, including night-lights with motion detectors.**
- **Check smoke and carbon monoxide alarms.**
- **Check all electrical cords for fraying and placement away from water or other hazards.**

Care Network

It is essential that you form a group of people who will visit and monitor your parent. It can include family members, friends, and neighbors. You need to monitor physical condition, food intake, liquid intake, and medical appointments. Keep a scale in their home; much information can be learned from their weight changes. When you call them, listen to the tone, words, and content. Elderly people who suffer from memory impairment will say the same thing more than once; even if what they are telling you sounds correct and in place, look for small changes in what they are communicating, not necessarily big changes.

Medication

You need to set up a simple way to remind your parents to take their medication (the right medication and on time) and verify that they do take their medications correctly (do not hesitate to count the pills). Weekly/daily pill boxes are available at any drugstore. Always keep an updated list of their medications with you. Remove any old, expired medications from their house. You just might find a 10-year-old medication in the medicine cabinet.

Mail

Filter their mail to remove all credit card applications, and donation requests. Elderly people are very vulnerable and there are many unscrupulous people who will take advantage of them.

Insurance

It is very important that you consult with your insurance agent to learn how to best protect your parent at home. Housekeepers/caregivers should be insured and bonded; if the caregiver is driving your parent(s) in your parents' car, make sure that the caregiver is put on their car insurance and you have a copy of his/her driving record.

Stimulation

While they are home, try to get them engaged in some outings, activities, Day Care, Senior Centers, etc.

While they are still in their home, take the time to prepare yourself for the next big bridge they will have to cross, moving from their home to a more secure environment (Rest Home, Nursing Home, etc.). Check to find what is available in your community. Visit the facilities, and ask a lot of questions. Participate in support groups, as you can learn a lot from other people's experiences. Be prepared.

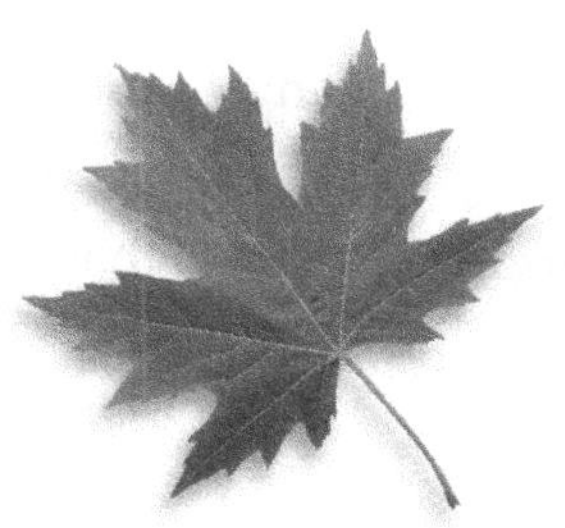

CHAPTER 21

Personality and Behavior Changes in the Elderly With Dementia

Some of the greatest challenges of caring for a loved one with dementia are the personality and behavior changes that often occur. You can best meet these challenges by using creativity, flexibility, patience, and compassion. It also helps to not take things personally and to maintain your sense of humor.

To start, consider these ground rules:

We cannot change the person. The person you are caring for has a brain disorder that shapes who he has become. When you try to control or change his behavior, you'll most likely be unsuccessful or be met with resistance. It is important to:

- Try to accommodate the behavior, not control the behavior. For example, if the person insists on sleeping on the floor, place a mattress on the floor to make him more comfortable.

- Remember that *we* can change our behavior or the physical environment. Changing our own behavior will often result in a change in our loved one's behavior.

Check with the doctor first. Behavioral problems may have an underlying medical reason: perhaps the person is in pain or experiencing an adverse side effect from medications. In some cases, like incontinence or hallucinations, there may be some medication or treatment that can assist in managing the problem.

Behavior has a purpose. People with dementia typically cannot tell us what they want or need. They might do something that we regard as unusual, such as take all the clothes out of the closet on a daily basis, and we wonder why. It is very likely that the person is fulfilling a need to be busy and productive. Always consider what need the person might be trying to meet with their behavior, and, when possible, try to accommodate them.

Behavior is triggered. It is important to understand that all behavior is triggered—it doesn't occur out of the blue. It might be something a caregiver or visitor did or said that triggered a behavior or it could be a change in the physical environment. The starting point for changing behavior is to disrupt the patterns that we create. Try a different approach, or try a different consequence.

What works today may not work tomorrow. The multiple factors that influence troubling behaviors and the natural progression of the disease process means that solutions that are effective today may need to be modified tomorrow—or may no longer work at all. The key to managing difficult behaviors is being creative and flexible in your strategies to address a given issue.

Get support from others. You are not alone—there are many others caring for someone with dementia. Call your local Area Agency on Aging, or the local chapter of the Alzheimer's Association, to find support groups, organizations, and services that can help you. Expect that, similarly to the loved one you are caring for, you will have good days and bad days. Develop strategies for coping with the bad days.

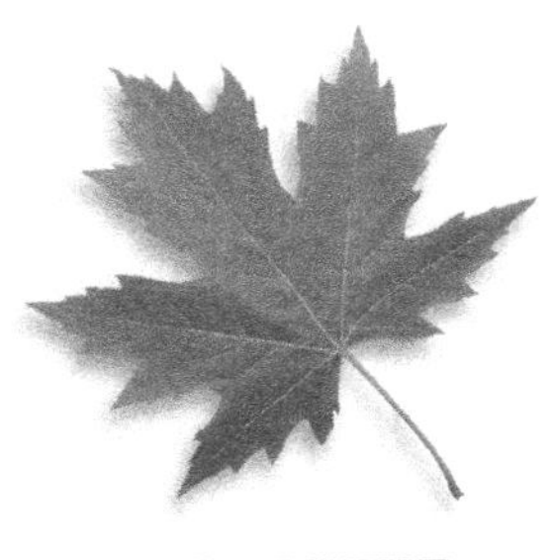

CHAPTER 22

Dementia and Urinary Incontinence

What is incontinence?

Incontinence is the loss of control of the bladder and/or bowel function. Our brains send messages to our bladder and bowel telling them when it is necessary to empty them. Being in control of these functions depends upon awareness of bodily sensations such as the feeling of having a full bladder, and the memory of how, when, and where to respond. When there is a decline of intellect and memory as a result of dementia, incontinence may occur.

Bladder control problems

Why do people with dementia experience bladder control problems?

People with dementia suffer memory loss and may be confused and disorientated. This can cause a breakdown in the mechanisms necessary for bladder control. Dementia causes changes in the brain which may interfere with their ability to:

- Recognize the need to pass urine;
- "Hold on" until they get to the toilet;
- Find the toilet;
- Recognize when the bladder is completely empty;
- Adjust clothing appropriately.

Incontinence may develop or worsen in unfamiliar surroundings, or during episodes of depression, anxiety, or stress.

Remember

People with dementia, just like other adults, are susceptible to other causes of incontinence such as urinary tract infection, constipation, atrophic vaginitis (vaginal irritation and inflammation after menopause), an enlarged prostate gland, or side effects of certain medications.

Can anything be done for dementia sufferers with incontinence? YES!

While their dementia may prevent them from participating in some treatments, much may be possible to ensure maximum comfort and dignity.

Seek help from their doctor who may be able to treat them directly or will refer them to a continence advisor for a continence assessment.

Management strategies

Assessment involves a physical examination and taking a history of relevant information. Difficulties encountered by the patient may include:

- Forgetting to take down clothes when going to the toilet;
- Having difficulty finding the toilet;
- Urinating in inappropriate places;
- Passing urine more often than usual;
- Saturating clothing/bedding without warning;
- Urinating with the action of standing up from a chair or bed;
- Suffering from constipation, or diarrhoea faecal incontinence.

Caring for someone with incontinence

When caring for someone with dementia, incontinence may seem like the last straw. But there are measures that can be taken to alleviate the problem itself or to make it less stressful. It is important for you to seek professional help at an early stage and not struggle on your own. Incontinence can be very distressing for the person with dementia. It helps if you, the caregiver, remain calm, gentle, firm, and patient, and try to accept and get over your own embarrassment in having to help the person in such an intimate way. Sometimes a little humor can help.

Information you need to collect for the doctor

It is useful if you can provide the doctor with the following information:

- How often is the person incontinent?

- Is it urinary and/or faecal incontinence?
- When did the problem start?
- Is the person saturating clothing or is it just a dribble?
- Has there been an increase in confusion or any change in behavior?
- Has there been any fever or does the person appear to find it painful to go to the toilet?
- Is the person taking any medication?
- Does the person pass urine in strange places (rather than in a bathroom)?

If medical assessment does not indicate that there are any other medical reasons for the incontinence, then the cause is most likely to be the person's dementia.

It is often necessary to rely on the caretaker to provide this important information and to record bladder and bowel function. That is:

- What time the person goes to the toilet and/or wets.
- How wet the person is, for example:

  minor = dampness in underpants;

  moderate = wets through to skirts/pants;

  severe = floods chair/floor/bed.
- How often they move their bowels.

What can be done to minimize the episodes of incontinence and maintain the person's dignity?

1. Underlying conditions such as urinary tract infection, constipation or atrophic vaginitis (inflammation of vagina and surrounding tissue after menopause) often respond to treatment and the incontinence may possibly subside.
2. In some situations, medications will help, but they can also worsen incontinence and increase confusion. Therefore, medications must be closely monitored and altered if any side effects occur.
3. Where possible, encourage the person to drink six to eight glasses of fluids a day, unless otherwise advised by their doctor. This helps to prevent urinary tract infection and constipation and to maintain good bladder health. Avoid excessive amounts of coffee, tea, and cola as the caffeine in these drinks may irritate the bladder and can cause frequency and urgency to pass urine.
4. Use good eating habits to maintain regular bowel habits; take necessary steps to prevent/treat constipation.
5. The person may need to be reminded to use the toilet at regular intervals, at the times when they usually need to go or before they are likely to be wet.
6. If they are no longer able to recognize the need to use the toilet, they should be taken to the toilet at regular intervals. This may be every two to three hours, depending on how much they drink and their urinating pattern. It may be necessary to stay with them in the bathroom, to help them and remind them why they are there. Frequent toileting (for example, hourly) is not encouraged.

7. Adjust clothing, if appropriate, to make it easier for them to manage. For example, use Velcro fastening instead of zippers and buttons; easy-to-manage clothing, such as tracksuits, may make undressing an easier task.
8. Keep the way to the toilet clear and free of clutter and use a night-light, if needed. Make the toilet door easily identifiable.
9. Whilst the above may or may not overcome the incontinence, such steps may reduce the incidence or severity of the problem. Quality of life for the person with dementia and the caregiver may also be improved by the use of incontinence aids such as pads. It may be possible to receive some financial assistance with the cost of incontinence aids.

Advice on eligibility and the types of aids available can be sought from:

- Your primary care physician
- Alzheimer's Foundation
- Needs Assessment Service coordinator
- Local hospital (check with Primary Care Physician)
- Elder services or council on aging in your area

Consider utilizing community resources to assist with the demands of caring for a person with dementia. Home Help or District Nursing may be available in the local area. Consult the patient's doctor or a continence advisor (through the patient's primary care physician) for help.

Can medication be helpful in treating the person with dementia and incontinence?

In the first instance, their doctor should review all medications being taken, as some of these may actually be causing or aggravating the incontinence. In some cases, medications can be prescribed by their doctor to help them overcome their incontinence. For example:

- Antibiotics may be prescribed to treat a recognized urinary tract infection. Be aware that most physicians are very concerned about the frequent use of antibiotics to treat urinary infections because of the possibility of infection with Clostridium difficile (klos-TRID-e-um dif-uh-SEEL). Often referred to as simply C-diff, C. difficile is a bacterium that can cause symptoms ranging from diarrhea to life-threatening inflammation of the colon. Illness from C. difficile most commonly affects older adults who are in hospitals or long-term care facilities, and typically occurs after use of antibiotic medications. However, studies indicate increasing rates of C. difficile infection among people traditionally not considered high risk, such as young and healthy individuals without a history of antibiotic use or exposure to healthcare facilities. Each year, more than a half million people get sick from C. difficile, and in recent years, C. difficile infections have become more frequent, severe, and difficult to treat.
- Hormone replacement therapy (tablets, patches, or vaginal creams) may help post-menopausal women by reducing frequency and urgency caused by atrophic vaginitis.

- Bladder relaxant tablets may be given to help calm an irritable bladder and thus improve its capacity. This may reduce the urgency and frequency of urination.
- Tablets may occasionally be given to help pass urine when there is an obstruction or blockage preventing discharge.

Be aware that these medications may produce side effects such as a dry mouth, constipation, impaired balance, and lethargy. In the person with dementia, there is also a risk of increased confusion. Medication use requires careful professional monitoring.

At the end of life, continence care should be based on the patient's wishes and preferences. This consensual approach ensures that care is given in a partnership of mutual respect and trust.

While continence care to the general population is aimed at promoting continence, the perspective may change in end-of-life care. Care is more often aimed at maintaining comfort and dignity and relieving symptoms with minimal interference. A good knowledge of urinary dysfunction is essential to inform the assessment of patients' needs.

Little is known about the continence needs of people as they near the end of their life and there is little evaluation of the approaches to managing their urinary continence needs. A collaborative approach among continence and palliative care health professionals would help to develop this important aspect of end-of-life care.

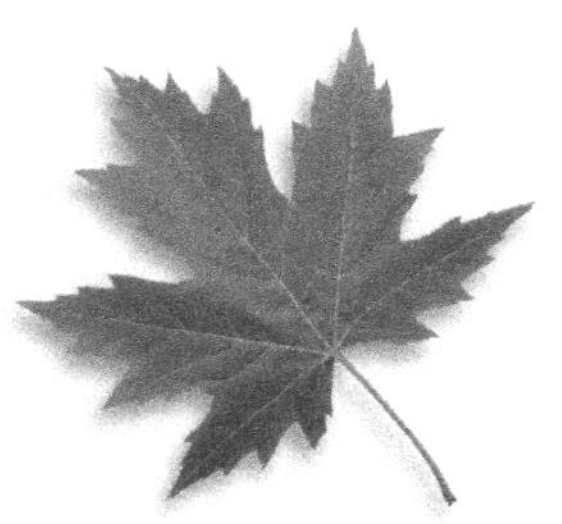

CHAPTER 23

Battle of the Shower/Bath With a Dementia Resident

I take care of my mother who has dementia. With bath, it's always a battle! I try to convince her that she needs a bath but she resists. She can't bathe herself anymore.

Professional and family caregivers often report bathing as one of the most challenging areas of dementia care. People with dementia virtually never worry about whether they look or smell good, and they often believe they have just recently had a bath—so why on earth should they take another one just because you think they need it? You may often find yourself having to get very creative about how to get them into the bathtub or shower.

There are many things that can trigger these unhealthy responses and many of these triggers can be controlled.

A certified nurse assistant (CNA) or family caregiver often does not have the advanced expertise to identify the trigger, devise a prevention strategy, or identify a helpful response. We must clearly document how the causative factor, which is the recurring problem behavior, impacts the person's level of independence and/or safety. Family members, physicians, therapists, and the facility management team (if the patient resides in a long-term care facility), should all be part of the professional team and should brainstorm together to find a positive approach to bath and shower time.

How to Identify the Behavior Trigger

It is critical to allocate some evaluation time to observation of the patient with the caregiver in the actual shower/bath environment. This is the only way that the trigger and other problems can be identified. In my experience, I have seen the following as common problem behaviors exhibited during the shower or bath experience:

- Physical resistance including hitting, pushing, kicking, and biting;
- Verbal agitation such as "leave me alone," crying out, yelling, or cursing;
- Withdrawal and fear in which the person may shake, cry, or hold themselves tightly and rock;
- Refusal.

Some likely causes/triggers include:

- Unmanaged pain
- Being cold
- Feeling frightened, vulnerable, and exposed

- Feeling embarrassed
- Feeling a loss of control
- Lack of understanding with regard to what is happening, misperceptions, and poor communication

I have found the following interventions to greatly reduce the frequency and severity of the behavior:

1. Reduce pain by:
    - Changing PRN (administered "as needed") pain medications to a routine schedule;
    - Making sure the body is positioned comfortably;
    - Providing a gentle touch.

2. Keep the person warm by:
    - Keeping the body covered as much and often as possible with warm towels;
    - Maintaining a comfortable temperature of both the room and the water;
    - Making sure the person is fully clothed or wearing a warm robe while moving to the shower/tub area.

3. Reduce fear by:
    - Increasing safety in the environment through the use of secure grab-bars, bath mats, or other non-skid surfaces. Make sure the person's feet are firmly placed on the floor and are not dangling.

- Building a relationship with the patient. Changes in caregivers should be minimal.
- Avoiding water spraying on the face, as the water spray can be painful or frightening for some people. Consider using non-rinse soaps.
- Making the shower/bathing environment look and feel homelike and inviting.
- Communicating what is about to happen during each step of the activity.
- Making the shower/bath fun or relaxing by setting the tone through music, lighting, addition of bubbles or candles, etc. (always remember safety needs and codes).
- Exercising patience. Wait the adequate amount of time for a patient to process and respond.

4. Reduce embarrassment by:
    - Keeping the body covered as much as possible.
    - Making certain the person feels safe and comfortable with you, the caregiver. For example, a caregiver of the opposite sex may upset a patient.

5. Maintain the patient's sense of control by:
    - Always asking for permission instead of saying, "It is time to take a shower."
    - Providing choices throughout the experience.

- Facilitating independence.
- Honoring the person's preferences for shower versus bath, products, time of day, etc. If the person is unable to communicate their needs and wants, gather their life story from other family members (or from any family member, if you are a hired caregiver).

6. Reduce the risk for misperceptions and miscommunication by:
   - Communicating what you are there to help the person with, and explaining what is going to happen throughout each step of the activity.
   - Recognizing the patient's current level of cognitive function. The Allen Battery comprises assessment tools and references, including the Allen Cognitive Level Screen (ACLS). The screening tools are designed to provide an initial estimate of cognitive function. The score from the screen must be validated by further observations of performance. The ACLS can help identify the Allen Cognitive Levels of clients with Alzheimer's disease, dementia, and other cognitive disabilities. For those who are lower functioning (Allen Level 3 or lower), consider using sensory bridging techniques such as providing a favorite/familiar soap or shampoo for the patient to smell before engaging the patient in the activity. This can help the patient connect to a memory related to the activity, and facilitate a higher level of understanding and independence.

- Using the proper cueing strategies and communication techniques to increase understanding; match these to the person's cognitive level.
- Closely observing the patient's responses and adjusting the approach as needed.

Ways to Focus on Positive Aspects

Two other care aspects that play a key role in directing the mood and behavior of the patient are: (1) promoting best ability to function, and (2) gaining agreement.

Promoting Best Ability to Function

Managing as much as possible of the bathing activity independently will provide a sense of control, accomplishment, and privacy to the patient. The therapist must alter the activity demands, environment, and care approach to facilitate the greatest degree of patient participation and independence. Caregivers should receive training in developing an activity modification plan until competency is achieved.

Gaining Agreement

The most effective method to reduce resistance or refusal is simply to gain agreement from the patient. This often requires the caregiver to be creative in finding an approach that might encourage patient agreement.

Examples include:

- Telling the patient they will/might have a family or clergy visit later in the day and therefore it would be nice to get freshened up.
- Taking the patient into the kitchen or garden, having fun, and getting obviously dirty. This blatant dirt can trigger the client to ask for the shower or bath.
- Honoring the preferences of the patient that are based upon their individual life story. For example, a patient might have always enjoyed a relaxing bath at night, and will, therefore, value the pleasure of bathing versus the task of getting clean.

Summary

Assisting a dementia patient with taking a bath or shower does not have to be a horrific experience. Remember that many of the behaviors are triggered. ALWAYS stop and ask yourself, "Would I be agreeable to bathing or showering at this time of day or in this environment or with this approach?" This perspective helps us to identify some of the changes that must be made. In addition, we must factor in all that we know about the patient's life story and cognitive level. Each has a direct relationship to the trigger management, prevention strategies, and environmental modifications that the therapist will design.

When you care for a person with dementia, you often find yourself deciding which battles you will fight. Bathing should not be one of them. If it is quite an accomplishment to manage a bath once weekly instead of twice, so be it. As the dementia progresses, something you attempted successfully a few months ago may not work well with them today. It becomes a game of constantly changing the rules, and the more flexible you are, the less stress you will feel. Try to keep in mind that one of the goals is to keep your stress level reduced, and the other goal is to keep your loved one clean and happy. In the grand scheme of things, missing a few baths is not a catastrophe, so try not to take on that stress.

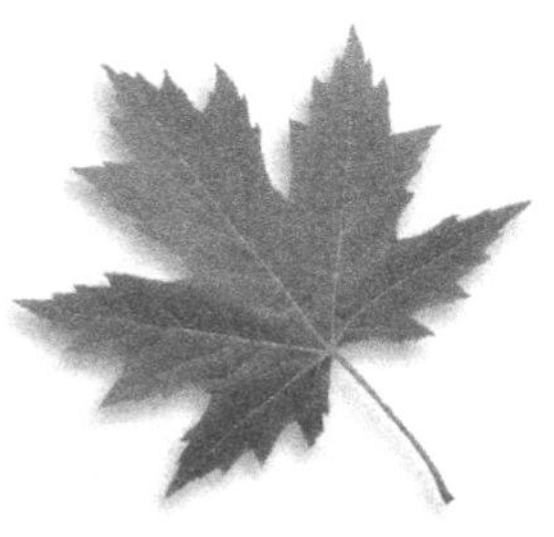

CHAPTER 24

Nutrition and Eating Patterns in Alzheimer's Disease Patients

There are many factors that interfere with food consumption and absorption among the population with Alzheimer's disease (AD). The person who lives alone may lack the cognitive resources to shop for, plan, and cook a nourishing meal. A loss of coordination may make it difficult to pick up utensils and to get food and drink to the mouth. Spilling food may embarrass the person in the early stages of AD. In the later stages, loss of oral control and hyperorality may make it difficult to get adequate nourishment.

Factors that potentially hinder proper eating and nutrition in AD patients may be assessed by considering the "As" of Alzheimer's:

- Aphasia: Difficulty articulating preferences orally
- Apraxia: Difficulty maneuvering food utensils, difficulty chewing and swallowing food
- Agnosia: Difficulty recognizing utensils and food

- Amnesia: May not remember eating or distinguishing the need to eat
- Anorexia: Decreased appetite (psychological cause possible)

Cognitive deficits related to short attention span, disorientation, and memory loss all contribute to the inability to complete a meal. The patient may hide food or throw it away, or may be unaware of or unable to respond to hunger and thirst sensations. Sensory-perceptual deficits interfere with eating skills. Those who have agnosia are not able to identify eating utensils, and may try to comb their hair with the fork. The patient with apraxia may know what the fork is and how to use it, but be unable to pick it up and bring food to the mouth. Some may perseverate during eating, chewing the same mouthful of food over and over. Others may tire of eating, or lose interest before the meal is completed.

Poor positioning also impedes the eating process. The table may be too high and the food too far away. Poor oral hygiene can predispose the patient to problems that cause loss of appetite, difficulty in chewing, and pain from oral lesions. In the later stages, dysphagia obstructs nutritional intake. The late-stage patient is unable to feed him or herself and may refuse to eat. Decisions should be made regarding aggressive nutrition and rehydration measures.

Food texture must be adapted to the diminishing skills. Barring other medical conditions, the patient can be placed on a regular diet, though one that still avoids tough, stringy meats and foods that are difficult to chew, such as caramels. A mechanically soft diet with ground or chopped foods may become necessary. Eventually, a pureed diet is usually required. Commercial thickeners added to fluids will facilitate swallowing.

Remember the old adage, you are what you eat? Make it your motto, because it is near to the truth.

Choosing a variety of colorful fruits and vegetables, whole grains, and lean proteins makes us feel vibrant and healthy, inside and out.

Live longer and stronger—good nutrition keeps muscles, bones, organs, and other body parts strong for the duration. Vitamin-rich foods boost immunity and fight illness-causing toxins. A well-rounded diet also reduces the risk of disease (e.g., heart disease, stroke, high blood pressure, type-2 diabetes, bone loss, cancer, and more). Additionally, eating sensibly means fewer calories and better weight management.

Brain power—key nutrients empower the brain to do its job. People who eat a wide variety of healthy foods, especially those packed with omega-3 fatty acids, improve focus and decrease the risk of dementia disease problems.

Feel better—wholesome meals give you more energy and help you feel better from the inside, out.

As we age, we can become healthy and stay healthy for years to come, by making healthy choices. A balanced diet and daily physical activity contribute to improved quality of life, and are the two lifestyle choices we have the most control over each and every day. Consider the following choices:

Fruit—Focus on whole fruits rather than fruit juice. Whole fruits have more fiber and vitamins, and older adults are said to need 1.5 to 2 servings daily.

Hint: The more color the better, and berries are especially good to include every day as they are full of antioxidants.

Veggies—Go for COLOR! Choose antioxidant-rich dark, leafy greens (e.g., kale, spinach, broccoli, etc.) as well as orange and yellow vegetables (e.g., carrots, squash, and yams). Older adults need 2 to 2.5 cups daily.

Calcium—Maintaining bone health through the aging process is vital. Adequate calcium is needed, which helps in the prevention of osteoporosis and bone fractures. Older adults need 1,200 mg of calcium daily, and ideally most of it comes from wholesome foods.

Grains—Be smart about your carbohydrates. Choose whole grains over processed white flour/high-sugar items for added nutrient density and fiber. To be sure, read the label to verify that the first word on the ingredient list is "whole." Your patient needs 6 to 7 ounces of grains daily.

Protein—Seniors need about 0.5 grams per pound of body-weight. Simply divide bodyweight in half to know how many grams are needed. A 130-pound woman will need about 65 grams of protein daily. A serving of tuna, for example, has about 40 grams of protein. Vary the source of protein by including other fish, as well as beans, peas, nuts, eggs, milk, cheese, and seeds.

Water—With age, the body becomes more prone to dehydration because it loses some of its ability to regulate fluids, and our sense of thirst becomes somewhat dulled. Have your care-recipient carry a water bottle (start with a 20-ounce and progress to a 32-ounce) around and have him pledge to drink two bottles daily. Your efforts will help your patient avoid urinary tract infections, constipation, and/or possible bouts of confusion.

Hints:

Thirst is a sign that we are already dehydrated.

Vitamin B. After 50, the stomach produces less gastric acid, which makes it more difficult to absorb vitamin B-12 (needed for vital blood and nerve-type function). The recommended daily intake of B-12 via fortified foods or a vitamin supplement is 2.4 mcg.

Vitamin D. Most of our vitamin D intake (essential for calcium absorption) comes through sun exposure and/or from specific foods (e.g., fatty fish, egg yolk, enriched milk, etc.). Aged skin becomes less efficient at synthesizing vitamin D. Consult the patient's doctor for specific suggestions regarding supplementation (e.g., fortified foods or a multivitamin).

Once we get used to the healthier options, our bodies rebel against various unhealthy choices by feeling slow and/or sluggish. The following suggestions will serve as a good start in your quest to create habits of healthy eating for both caregiver and care-receiver:

1. Reduce your sodium (salt) to help prevent water retention and high blood pressure.

   Look for the "low sodium" label and season with spices instead of salt. Enjoy the good fats; monounsaturated fats such as olive oil, avocados, salmon, walnuts, and flaxseed are "good." The fat from these delicious sources serves to raise HDLs/good cholesterol levels while lowering LDLs/bad cholesterol levels.

2. Add fiber. Avoid constipation, lower the risk of chronic diseases, and feel fuller longer by increasing your fiber

intake (e.g., fresh fruits and vegetables, whole grains, and beans).

3. Avoid the bad carbohydrates. Bad carbs (simple or unhealthy carbs) are generally white-based foods (e.g., white flour, white sugar, white rice, white pasta, etc.). These foods have been stripped of all bran, fiber, and nutrients. Bad carbs digest quickly, cause a spike in blood sugar, produce short-lived energy and lead to weight gain. For the opposite results (e.g., long-lasting energy, stable blood sugars, etc.) opt for complex/good carbs (e.g., whole grains, beans, fruits, and vegetables.
4. Watch for hidden sugar. Added sugar is everywhere in a variety of foods (e.g., breads, canned soups and vegetables, pasta sauces, instant mashed potatoes, frozen dinners, fast food, ketchup, peanut butter, and more). Read labels and know terms, other than sugar, that constitute the same thing (e.g., corn syrup, molasses, brown rice syrup, cane juice, fructose, sucrose, dextrose, or maltose). Opt for fresh or frozen vegetables instead of canned, and choose low-carb or sugar-free options (e.g., tortillas, bread, pasta, etc.).
5. Cook conscientiously. Optimal preparation of vegetables is steaming or sautéing in an effort to preserve nutrients. Note that boiling drains nutrients from vegetables. Create a colorful platter. Understand that the more color you see on your plate, the richer the levels of vitamins, minerals, and nutrients.

Remember, variety is the spice of life! Inspire new ideas for eating healthy by going to your local farmers' market, browsing through healthy cooking magazines, buying something new and healthy each time you shop, trying a food/spice you haven't tried before, or chatting with friends about their personal health food options.

By making variety a priority, you will find it easier to get creative as you eat/cook your way to improved health and wellness. Be healthy … be happy!

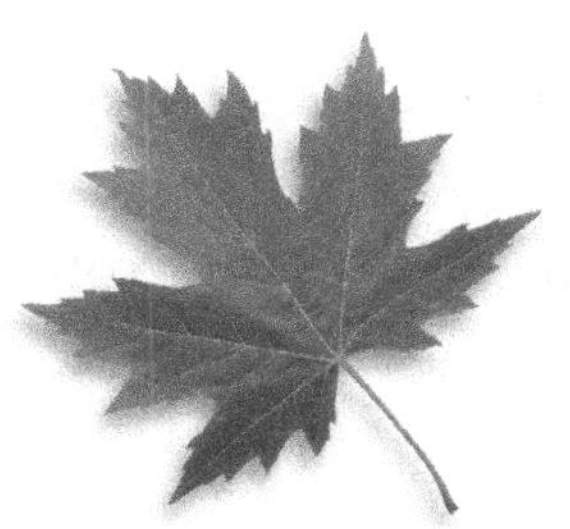

CHAPTER 25

Alzheimer's Care at Home: A Little-Known Secret Regarding the High Cost Associated With It

Over 35 million people worldwide will eventually forget the names of their children, spouses, and friends. And those forgotten will witness with sadness and frustration as the Alzheimer's disease slowly steals away the loved one they once knew. Alzheimer's disease and related dementias affect an alarming number of individuals across the globe, creating one of the most significant social and health crises of the 21st century.

Who will provide Alzheimer's care to the patient?

In most families, a dilemma comes into play very quickly. Can we afford to pay for outside services, and if not, can we risk the health of the patient if we become the primary caregiver in a stressful and difficult situation? While having family members become the caregiver for a loved one eliminates the cost of an outside care provider, there will be other hidden costs associated with the arrangement.

It is often helpful for caregivers to know they are not alone. Given the prevalence of Alzheimer's disease, many caregivers find themselves in situations similar to others, trying to balance work and family life while also caring for an aging parent or other relative.

Some pertinent facts from the *2010 Alzheimer's Disease Facts and Figures*:

- A typical Alzheimer's family caregiver is a woman between 50 and 64 years of age, who works full or part time.
- Most Alzheimer's caregivers (94 percent) are helping relatives. The most common caregiving relationship is between a parent or parent-in-law and child (62 percent).
- An estimated 10.9 million family members and friends provided unpaid care for a person with Alzheimer's disease or another dementia in 2009, each providing an average of 21.9 hours of care per week.
- An estimated 0.9 to 1.6 million caregivers of people with Alzheimer's and other dementias are "long-distance caregivers," living more than an hour away.

A new study puts the cost of treating Alzheimer's and other forms of dementia at $109 billion, making it more expensive to society than either cancer or heart disease.

This study, which appeared in the *New England Journal of Medicine*, also estimates that costs of treatment will more than double in the next 27 years, reaching $259 billion by 2040. The same study puts the estimated cost of treating heart disease at $102 billion, and cancer treatment at $77 billion.

The cost of formal care comes to a yearly average of $33,329 for each patient with dementia. Both the average annual cost of care, and the number of patients suffering from dementia, are forecast to rise in coming years.

The media often writes about the high cost of long-term care, but often overlooks the even higher cost of home care that is instead provided by family caregivers. Let's look at some of the areas that account for the costs to family caregivers:

1. Absenteeism from gainful employment largely as a result of workday interruptions, such as a crisis in care, or supervision of care;
2. Loss of all sick days and vacation days, and having to request unpaid leave;
3. Loss of wages during unpaid leave;
4. Loss of wages when work hours are reduced from full-time to part-time;
5. Loss of wages when status changes from part-time to unemployed, to allow 24/7 shifts in the home;
6. Cost for a mental health provider to support (via visits or meds) and help the caregiver with the stress of the daily living and caregiving.

Most people probably wouldn't anticipate the cost of the caregiver's health: taking care of a family member with Alzheimer's disease could make your own healthcare bills increase by an average of $4,766 per year. Family caregivers make visits to emergency rooms, doctors, and hospitals at higher rates than other people the same age. Those costs add up, according to research released by the National Alliance for Caregiving, an advocacy group presenting at the Gerontological Society of America's annual conference in Boston in 2012. The study looked specifically at formal health services used by a large swath of caregivers over an 18-month period.

Caring for a family member with such a personality-draining disease can take a hefty financial and emotional toll. Nearly 15 million people fall into the role of unpaid caregivers for those who are ill with dementia, according to the Alzheimer's Association. Added together, the total for this commitment was about 17 billion hours of unpaid care, which are valued at $202 billion in 2010 alone.

So to help with the staggering cost of care, the Obama administration included $26 million in the proposed 2013 budget. The money was designated for education, outreach, and support for families affected by the disease. It is not enough to solve the long-term care crisis in America, but it is a good start. More resources, and thinking outside the box, will be required in years to come.

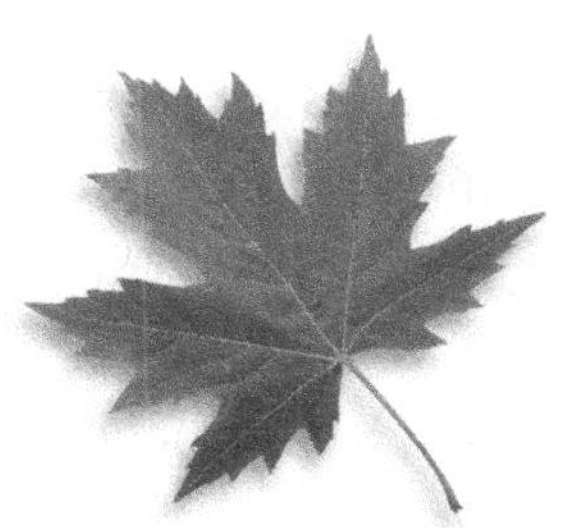

CHAPTER 26

Taking Care of You, the Caregiver!

By the year 2030, an estimated 20 percent of the U.S. population will be 65 years or older. As the American population ages, a growing number of people will be serving as caregivers for family members affected by dementia and other types of functional impairment. Dementia is present in 10 percent of individuals older than 65 years and in 47 percent of those older than 85 years.

Caregiving is such a small and innocent word for such a large and often stressful job.

While many understand that caring for someone with memory impairment can be physically, mentally, and emotionally exhausting, few realize that they could be putting their own health at risk. A study of elderly spouse caregivers, aged 66 to 96, found that caregivers who experience mental or emotional strain have a 63 percent higher risk of developing life-threatening health problems than do non-caregivers of the same age.

There are many terms used to describe well-being. Should you look the term up in the dictionary, you will find definitions including contentment, happiness, health, prosperity, and wellness. Well-being is a state of balance or harmony. Each of the dictionary terms, in reality, is an adjective that describes well-being. The definition of well-being is actually very personal, and also changeable. Events, situations, and circumstances that occur in one's life upset the balance within us and produces stress. Not everyone responds to life events with the same thoughts, feelings, and reactions. When we perceive life events to be stressful, or we exceed our stress threshold, it is not uncommon to experience *anxiety.* If we think of being in balance as "being in the present with oneself," then the anxiety-induced disruption of balance can result in feeling "ahead of oneself," worrying about what is to come, or "behind oneself," worrying about what has occurred. Finding ways to manage responses to stress is critical to well-being and maintaining one's personal balance. Developing your own foundation for well-being can help you, not only to find and promote your own balance, but to support well-being in the face of ongoing or increasing challenges that may be presented to you in your demanding role as caregiver.

Most of the research on the health of caregivers has focused on psychological well-being. Depression is the most heavily researched area in caregiver health. One study revealed that anxiety was present in 17.5 percent of caregivers, compared with 10.9 percent of subjects in a matched control group. Research has documented that the increased incidence of anxiety correlates with a higher amount of psychotropic drug use among caregivers.

Understandably, caregivers are often so concerned with care for their relative's needs, that they lose sight of their own well-being. Ignoring the signs of stress on the body can be both unhealthy and dangerous.

Fortunately, there are many resources available to assist caregivers. One tool offered by the Alzheimer's Association is self-assessment quizzes for you to evaluate your own stress level and risk factors. ***The best way to take care of others is to take care of you.*** You can be one less thing they have to worry about.

Please give yourself a gift today: log into the Alzheimer's Stress Check Site at http://alz.org/stresscheck/overview.asp?type=homepage and start taking good care of YOU!

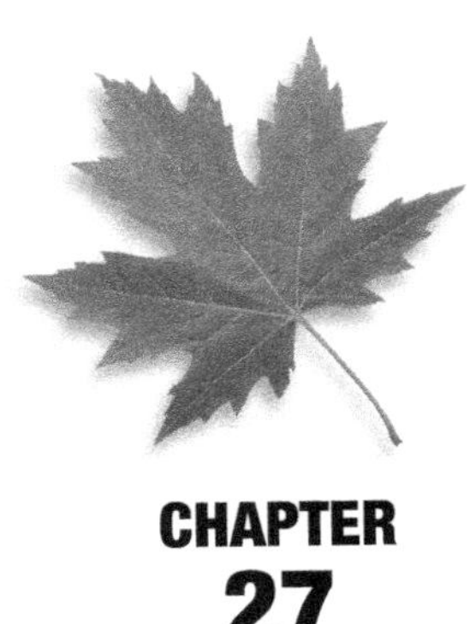

CHAPTER 27

Why Use Respite Care?

While being a family caregiver is a fulfilling role, it is also one that can consume a great deal of physical, mental, and emotional energy. Consequently, respite care is very important, because it gives family caregivers of persons with Alzheimer's and related dementia disease an opportunity to create a plan of care for themselves; this is something caregivers often overlook.

Respite care simply means an interval of rest or relief. Respite care gives you, the family caregiver, an opportunity to take a much-needed break from the daily care that you provide for your loved one. A period of respite may be a few hours or a few days at a time, depending on what is decided between you and the care-recipient. There are a number of ways you can spend your "time off" during your respite. Here are just a few examples:

- Go to the movies.
- Read a book at a nearby park.

- Go on a short vacation.
- Have someone else care for your loved one while you retreat to another part of the house and watch TV, read a book, or take a nap.
- Attend a caregiving support group.
- Sit in the sun.
- Take a walk.
- Treat yourself to lunch at a restaurant with a friend.
- Get a massage/facial/manicure ... do something for YOU.

It is important to have a plan for your own self-care because doing so can enhance the quality of life for you and the quality of life for your loved one. The more relaxed and fulfilled you feel, the more easily you will be able to provide the necessary care for your loved one. It is also possible that your loved one will appreciate a respite from the normal routine of care as well.

The lack of a conscious plan of self-care can result in caregiver burnout. How do you know if you are burning out? Some symptoms of caregiver burnout are:

- Social withdrawal
- Exhaustion
- Inability to concentrate or to relax
- Depression
- Inability to sleep
- Anxiety

- Irritability
- Forgetfulness
- Lack of appetite

Caregiver burnout makes the task of caregiving very difficult, if not impossible. It can lead to resentment on the part of the caregiver, and even illness. It is your responsibility, as a caregiver, to care for yourself as well as the person for whom you are providing care.

Respite care is one tool you can use to help yourself avoid caregiver burnout. To begin taking advantage of the benefits of receiving a reprieve from the routine care you provide to your loved one, follow the three steps below:

Step 1: Are you a family caregiver?

The first step to receiving help is to identify whether or not you are a family caregiver. Not everyone considers the care they provide to their loved one as "caregiving." However, you are indeed a family caregiver if you provide care to an ill family member such as assisting with areas of personal care, emotional support and companionship, finances, and maintaining the household.

Step 2: Have you discussed your needs with your loved one?

It is important to communicate your needs and desires with your loved one, the person you are providing care for. If you believe that you might like to pursue respite care services, it is essential to discuss this with your loved one. In doing so, you may discover that your loved one is very supportive of the idea. You may also find that having such a conversation opens up doors for even more communication and intimacy.

Step 3: How do you find out about respite services available to you?

Respite care can take different forms. In-home respite care usually involves a trained professional (often from a home health agency) who comes into the home to provide necessary care during a period of time when the caregiver is away.

Another way to partake in respite care services is through a facility or residence that employs trained health care staff on-site. This type of respite would allow your loved one to stay at such a residence on a short-term basis (as determined by you and your loved one) and entitle him or her to receive whatever care he or she needs.

A less formal way of receiving respite care assistance is by utilizing family and friends who are eager to be helpful. The next time a friend or family member asks you how they can help, consider responding by telling them that giving you a break for the day, an evening, or even for a few hours might be the nicest gift they can give to you.

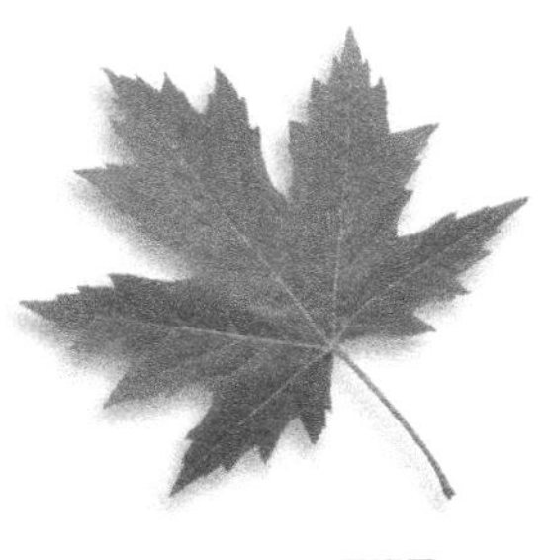

CHAPTER 28

How Do I Choose the Right Adult Day Care Program?

No matter how efficiently and effortlessly you have adapted your life to the role of caregiver, eventually you are going to need a break. Occasional breaks are essential, not only to your emotional well-being, but to the well-being of your relationships with your family, friends, and the person you are caring for. Taking an occasional break is also essential to maintaining your capability as a caregiver. For some caregivers, a nearby family member can step in and provide the care, but for other caregivers that option is not available. In those cases, adult day care is one option.

The role of adult day care is gaining increased attention as the nation prepares for the large cohort of baby boomers entering their later years. Many boomers are aging with physical and cognitive impairments, including Alzheimer's disease and related dementias. Moreover, these boomers have a strong preference to age in place in their communities. It is estimated that 70 percent of persons with dementia and Alzheimer's disease reside at home while receiving care from family members.

Life, liberty, and the pursuit of happiness are central ideals in American society. Health and aging issues in the United States are shaped by "independence, autonomy, the application of principles, and a preeminent concern for individual rights." In the United States, the National Adult Day Services Association (NADSA) provides leadership in all areas of Adult Day Services (ADS). The most current definition for ADS in the United States comes from the NADSA Standards and Guidelines for ADS:

> "Adult day services are community-based group programs designed to meet the needs of adults with impairments through individual plans of care. These structured, comprehensive, residential programs provide a variety of health, social, and related support services in a protective setting. By supporting families and other caregivers, adult day services enable participants to live in the community. Adult day services assess the needs of participants and offer services to meet those needs. Participants attend on a planned basis."

The Components of a Quality Program

Family members must do some research to determine whether the adult day care center is right for their loved one(s). The components of a quality adult day care program should include the following:

- Conducts an individual needs assessment before admission to determine the person's range of abilities and needs;
- Provides an active program that meets the daily social and recreational needs of the person in care;

- Develops an individualized treatment plan for participants and monitors it regularly, adjusting the plan as necessary;
- Has clear criteria for service and guidelines for termination based on the functional status of the person in care;
- Provides a full range of in-house services, which may include transportation, meals, health screening and monitoring, educational programs and counseling;
- Provides a safe, secure (locked if needed) environment;
- Provides transportation.

For each program you are considering, be sure to ask which services are included, and whether or not supplemental services may be purchased to complement the specific care and services required.

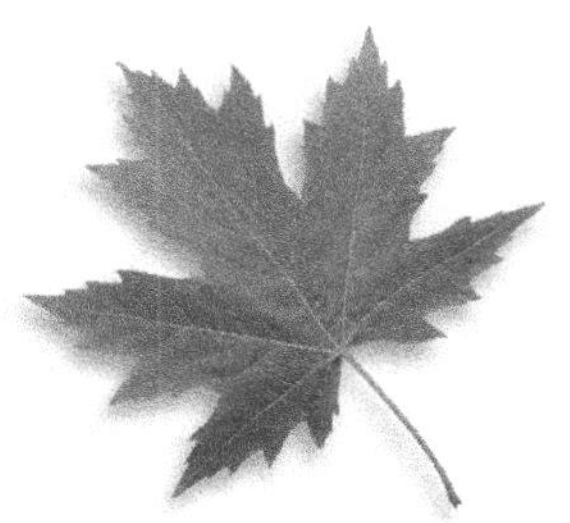

CHAPTER 29

Understanding the Help You Need as a Caregiver

About 44 million people, roughly 19 percent of the U.S. adult population, provide unpaid care to someone who is age 50 or older. The average age of caregivers is 50 and the average age of care-recipients is 77. Most caregivers assist family members, usually their mothers.

How do you define the term "caregiver" in less than a thousand words? Consider one especially telling statistic: more than 4 in 10 caregivers said they felt as though they had no choice about whether or not to assume the role of caregiver.

Why is it so hard to ask for help? What is a good response to the statement, "Call me if you need me"? Despite the fact that family caregivers are drowning in responsibility, or are really confused about what the next step ought to be, they often respond "No thanks" when help is offered. The following are steps to take in reaching out to those who can help:

1. Recognize that caregiving, like any job, is made up of lots

of individual tasks, not all of which are of the same importance. Some tasks take a few minutes, and some may take many hours. Some tasks are easy, while others require some skill and fortitude. The challenge is to know the difference.

2. Recognize that asking for help is a sign of strength and not of weakness. It means you truly have a grasp of your situation and have come up with a proactive problem-solving approach to making things easier and better.

3. Create a list of the tasks that need to get done in any given week, or at least those you are most concerned about, such as balancing your responsibilities at work with taking Mom or Dad to the doctor and Susie or Karen to soccer practice, or bathing and dressing your husband while providing cooking, cleaning, etc. When you see how long the list is, you'll quickly understand why you are so tired and don't have time for yourself.

4. Group your tasks into categories such as personal care tasks for your loved one, transportation, and household chores. You can group your tasks into only a few broad categories, or many specific ones. There's no right or wrong way to complete this task. It is all a matter of personal preference.

5. Write down your caregiving worries. Where will we get the money to pay for Peter's medications? Who will care for Mary if I get sick? Where can I find a day care facility that provides transportation? Seeing them in black and white helps diffuse some of the emotion attached to the questions. It also allows you to think more rationally about

your concerns and understand how getting help with some of your tasks might lessen the stress. It can provide the basis for deciding which tasks you might ask a neighbor, family member, or the church to help out with, which ones you are willing and able to pay someone else to do, and for which ones there might be a public program ready to provide assistance.

6. Share your lists with someone you trust before you actually reach out for help—a friend, therapist, professional care manager, or clergyman, perhaps. The intent is to first get comfortable with the idea of talking about your need for assistance, and hopefully get some encouragement and good ideas in the process. Then take a deep breath and actually ask someone to help with one of the tasks on your list, or ask for guidance in resolving your most persistent worry. Start with something small, especially if you are looking for hands-on assistance or something that requires someone doing you a favor.

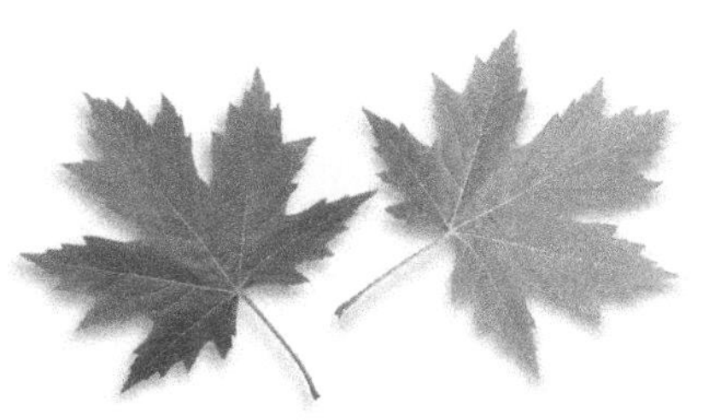

PART III
Long-Term Care Facilities

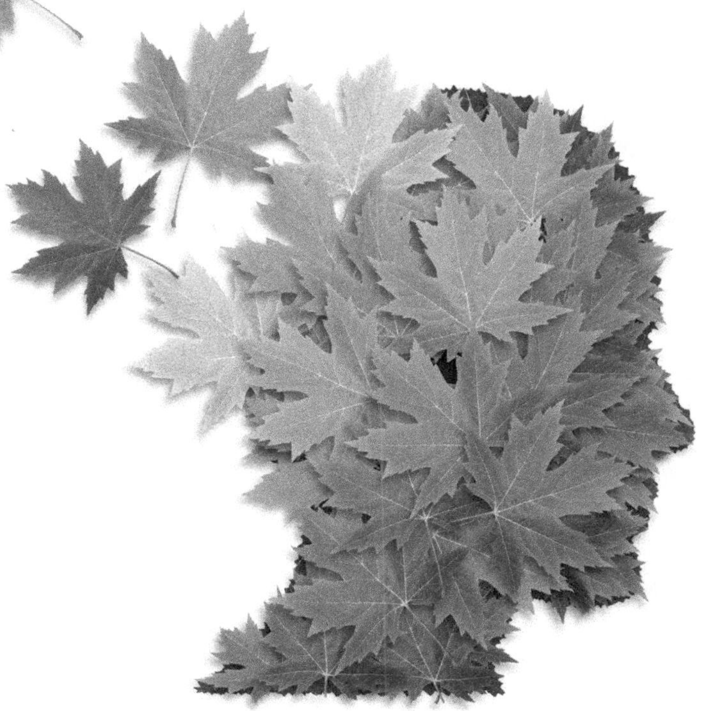

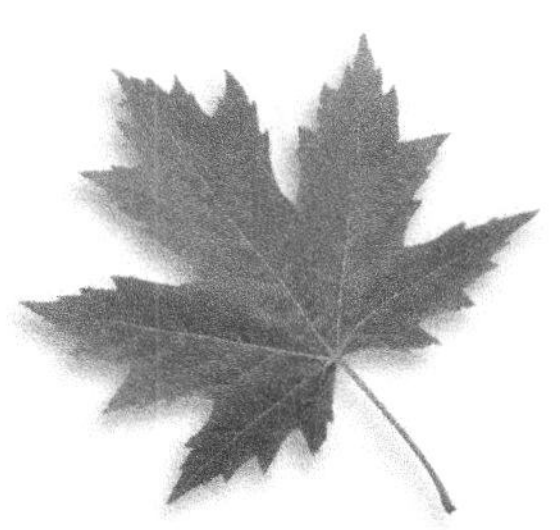

CHAPTER 30

When is the Right Time to Place a Loved One Who Suffers From Dementia in a Long-Term Care Facility?

The mid-stage of Alzheimer's/Dementia requires twenty-four-hour care. This may be the point when you consider institutionalization. To determine when you should place your loved one who suffers from Alzheimer's disease or dementia into a facility, consider two factors: your own physical and mental state, and your loved one's physical and mental state.

Your physical and mental state

For many caregivers, the time to place the elder in a facility is the point at which they themselves can no longer cope with the physical or mental demands of caregiving. If you are having coping difficulties, try various support services. Warning signs of the need for caregiver support are:

- Feeling very stressed, anxious, depressed, easily angered, or irritable
- Feeling exhausted or having sleep problems

- Deteriorating health
- Denial of depression observed by others
- Social withdrawal
- Loss of ability to concentrate

You can try to resolve these problems through a doctor, counselor, or Alzheimer's support group. Studies have shown that the more support and counseling a caregiver gets, the longer the resident stays at home.

The elder's mental and physical state

Some key behaviors or conditions in the resident that would cause you to consider a facility are:

1. The person is so physically abusive that you don't feel safe anymore.
2. The person wanders from home and jeopardizes his/her own safety.
3. The person requires constant medical/mental supervision.

At first consider adult day care or respite care to give yourself a break. Such a break may give you what you need to continue with caregiving for a while, or you may use the break to think more clearly about care in a facility for your loved one. Note that placing your relative who has dementia into a facility, may bring on added emotional stress. When caregivers place their loved one in a facility, they sometimes merely trade the stress of caring for a dementia resident for the stress of managing and witnessing care in a facility, at least for a while. On the other hand, a facility setting, in most situations, is better for the resident. It can be a good alternative to the isolation of home care, with the advantages of social stimulation and professional care.

Best types of facilities for Alzheimer's residents

Some facilities claim to specialize in treating the elder with Alzheimer's disease or other dementia, but not all of them excel in this kind of care. Those that do excel tend to be very expensive. If you cannot afford such care, look for a facility where you and others can visit frequently and assist with your loved one's needs. Ideally you'll find a facility where the following criteria are met:

Criteria for a good Alzheimer's care facility

- Caregivers help residents get ample movement. If the resident can move on their own, caregivers may need only to help the person get out of bed. Otherwise, caregivers will move the person within their bed and around the facility, including outdoors.
- Look for the smile. Do the staff members seem to be happy and enjoy what they are doing? This is a good indicator of the overall organizational health.
- It is best to have caregivers who interact with the resident in the resident's own language. Many residents revert to their native language in the later stages of Alzheimer's, and caregivers must adjust accordingly. Check for cultural sensitivity in how personnel care for residents.
- Dementia residents should be cared for together with other residents in a group setting. Studies have shown that the social aspects of a group are beneficial to residents with Alzheimer's or other dementias.

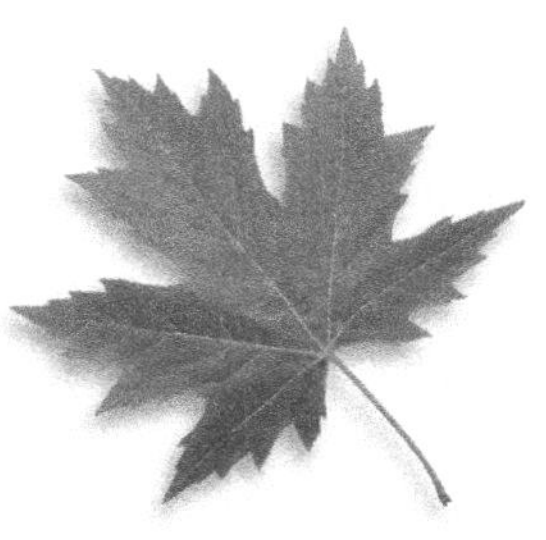

CHAPTER 31

"Aging in Place" Concept for Individuals Diagnosed With Dementia/Alzheimer's Disease

The phrase "home is where the heart is" captures the sentiments of many older adults when it comes to making choices about where they live as they age. Eighty-nine percent of those people 50 and over, who were surveyed in 2005, stated that they would prefer to remain in their home indefinitely as they age. Should they find themselves unable to do so, almost 85 percent of respondents agreed with the statement, "What I'd really like to do is remain in my local community for as long as possible."

Social connections with friends and neighbors, familiarity with local amenities, and proximity to services and even doctors, are among the many things that may be lost when an older adult has to move from his or her community.

While steps are being taken to make Aging in Place easier, the real challenge is answering "What strides are required for Aging in Place to reach its promise, and what level of care can be provided at a facility level to fully embrace the concept?"

As we age, health problems tend to be episodic, chronic, and sometimes progressive, resulting in an increasing need for assistance. Most ordinary "service-enriched" rest homes, nursing homes, assisted living and independent living communities are organized to provide care at a certain level of need, sometimes too much or too little for a particular individual. As a result, a housing arrangement often becomes a poor match, requiring residents to move multiple times, until the proper level of care is found.

When dealing with individuals with dementia and Alzheimer's disease, the situation is much more complicated. Moving between facilities is often disorienting, disturbing, and undesirable, not only for the individual, but for the entire family.

The process of selecting the right facility for your loved one's long-term care can be a difficult one. Often the decision needs to be made quickly, and occurs within the context of strong emotions, such as guilt, fear, and doubt.

Long-term facilities must respect the independence and judgment of residents. Aging in Place is a concept dedicated to maintaining and supporting independent living as long as possible. This model encourages a host of community services and resources to support seniors. Not only is Aging in Place a cost-effective way to manage the upcoming surge of seniors needing such services, it also supports what many seniors want most: living in the least restrictive environment as well as residing in a facility where they can wake up late, take showers as often as they wish, receive visitors any time during the day, host a child or a friend for a lunch or dinner, and feel free to engage in activities.

I would contend that the very word "place" (in the Aging-In-Place concept) is the root cause of much of the confusion and the reason many communities use this as more of a public relations "gimmick." By its very nature, it implies one's "house"—the place where we raised the kids, shared family experiences, and ventured from when wanting to walk the neighborhood. I propose that we change its definition.

Aging in Place should have nothing to do with physical location. It should have everything to do with self-fulfillment and personal empowerment. Aging in Place reflects an attitude and a way of environmentally enhancing the ability of seniors to maintain personal control over their lives, to the extent that is practical; retaining some control is important to them, regardless of the fact that they are suffering from dementia and/or Alzheimer's disease.

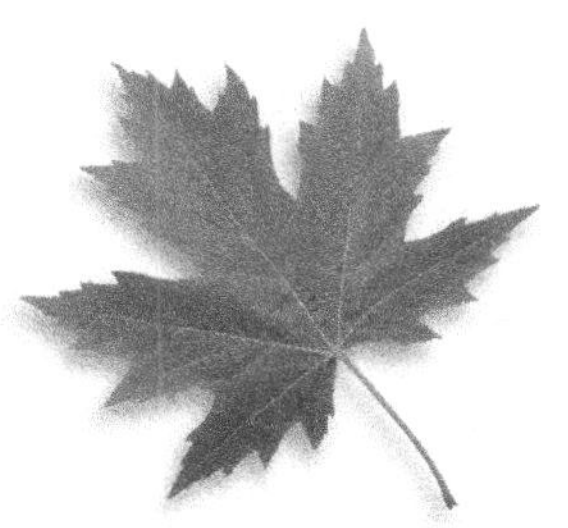

CHAPTER 32

Improving Dementia and Alzheimer's Care Through Individualized Care From a Medical Perspective

We begin to develop individual patterns of behavior at birth. Generally we know what others mean by listening to what they say and watching what they do. In the absence of verbal communication, we possess the ability to understand through other means, what others are communicating to us. If we lose the ability to speak, our actions become our method of communication.

In the United States, 25.2 percent of nursing facility residents receive antipsychotic medications (although this trend is in declining mode as per new report in 2013), according to data from the Online Survey Certification and Reporting Database (OSCAR), from the Centers for Medicare and Medicaid Services (CMS). In a survey of more than 4,000 nursing home residents in eight European countries (http://biomedgerontology.oxfordjournals.org/content/67A/6/698.abstract), the rate of antipsychotic drug use was even a little higher (26.4 percent).

In the nursing facility resident population, antipsychotics are generally used for three purposes:

1) Treatment of psychotic disorders (e.g., schizophrenia);
2) Treatment of psychotic symptoms (e.g., delusions and hallucinations) associated with other conditions (e.g., Alzheimer's disease or delirium);
3) Treatment of behavioral and psychological symptoms associated with dementia (BPSD), when these symptoms present a risk of harm to the resident or others.

Antipsychotics are also occasionally used for other purposes, such as in conjunction with an antidepressant in the treatment of refractory depression.

More than half of nursing home and assisted living residents have different forms of dementia, and many of these residents experience behavioral and psychological symptoms associated with dementia (BPSD). The preferred therapies for management of these symptoms are non-pharmacological, and include environmental modifications. If an underlying cause or reason for the behaviors can be identified, a non-pharmacological approach that addresses this underlying cause can be effective and safe.

In February 2012, the American Health Care Association announced a new, three-year quality initiative to help nursing homes and assisted living communities improve person-centered care for their residents. One of the goals of the initiative was to reduce the off-label use of antipsychotics by 15 percent by December 2012.

The American Society of Consultant Pharmacists has developed a Question and Answer document (PDF) on the use of antipsychotic medications in nursing facility residents. This 12-page document includes references to journal articles and useful Web sites (https://www.ascp.com/sites/default/files/ASCP-QnA-AntipsychoticsFinal.pdf).

On March 29, 2012, the Centers for Medicare and Medicaid Services released a webinar, "Initiative to Improve Behavioral Health and Reduce the Use of Antipsychotic Medications in Nursing Home Residents." This is the direct link to the site: http://surveyortraining.cms.hhs.gov/pubs/VideoInformation.aspx?cid=1098.

When we understand what residents are communicating, we can meet their needs instead of escalating their sense of crisis. For instance, agitation means "Help Me!" while aggression means "STOP!" Recognizing the meaning behind behaviors and using organizational practices, such as consistent staff assignment, can help staff build the relationships with residents that are necessary for them to understand and respond to this communication.

Behavioral symptoms, referred to as the secondary manifestation of the disease process, are common in individuals with dementia, and can occur throughout the course of the disease. Most individuals with dementia manifest at least one or more behavioral symptoms, with agitated-type behaviors being the most typical. Behavioral symptoms have a profound effect on individuals with dementia and their family members: compromised life quality, heightened caregiver burden and risk for nursing home placement, increased time spent in caregiving, and increased dollars spent in caregiver healthcare costs. Even passive behaviors (such as withdrawal and apathy) are reported by families to be sources of great frustration and sadness.

In the therapeutic context, common behavioral symptoms may include resistance, verbal or physical aggressiveness, agitation, and refusal to engage in the therapeutic session. To help patients achieve rehabilitative goals, it is important to understand why such behaviors may occur and identify ways to minimize or manage them.

The etiology of dementia-related behaviors and their relationship to the underlying pathology is still unclear. Although some studies show that the prevalence and severity of behaviors increase with global severity of dementia, other studies suggest a non-linear pattern with the most disturbing behaviors (aggressiveness) occurring at the moderate stage of the disease and diminishing with disease progression (McCarty et al., *Journal of Gerontology* 2000, 55[4]:M200; Gitlin et al., *Clinical Interventions in Aging* 2007, 2[4]:695). Nevertheless, research suggests that behavioral symptoms cannot be explained solely by diminished cognitive capacity. Rather, behaviors may reflect the interplay or interaction between the pathology, a person's capabilities, and the physical and social environment in which behaviors occur.

Efforts to manage behaviors, particularly hallucinations/delusions, agitation, and aggressiveness, typically have involved pharmacological treatments, specifically the off-label use of atypical antipsychotic drugs. Yet, these pharmacological approaches have been shown to yield only modest benefit, and at considerable cost. Recent evidence has led the Federal Drug Administration (FDA) to enforce a black box warning, requiring that manufacturers state that these medications may cause death in the elderly with dementia. There is also emerging evidence that non-pharmacological treatments compare favorably, even when a pharmacological solution exists. While a pharmacological approach may help manage certain psychiatric behaviors (e.g., hallucinations, paranoia, or mood disorders such as depression), common behavioral disturbances that occur in the therapeutic context or at home with families, such as wandering, resistance, agitation, or repetitive vocalizations, are much less amenable to drug management. Thus, there is considerable, and increasing, interest in the potential of non-pharmacological interventions. Recent consensus and white paper reports from organizations such as the American Association for Geriatric Psychiatry, The American Society of Neuropsychopharmacology, and the 2006 Geriatric Mental Health Expert Panel, have recommended that non-pharmacological approaches serve as the initial treatment of choice, prior to considering drug therapies (American Association of Geriatric Psychiatry 2005; American Psychiatric Association Work Group on Alzheimer's Disease and other Dementias 2007; Lyketsos et al., *American Journal of Geriatric Psychiatry* 2006, 14[7]:561; Salzman et al., *Journal of Clinical Psychiatry* 2008, 69[6]:889).

The patient with Moderate Dementia is impacted in behavioral aspects in the following ways:

- Experiences difficulties with short- and long-term memory;
- Struggles to learn new things;
- Experiences difficulties with understanding and being understood;
- Cannot self-regulate emotions;
- Is frequently and easily upset or frustrated;

- Can become fearful;
- May misinterpret the actions of others.

The patient with Severe Dementia is impacted in behavioral aspects in the following ways:

- Has limited/no short- and long-term memory, and therefore often lives in the moment;
- Cannot learn new information or pick up new routines;
- Is unable to carry on meaningful conversation;
- May appear withdrawn and can have difficulty interacting or responding to surroundings.

In short—what we label as "behavior" in dementia is really a method of communication by the person affected. Our job is to figure that out and respond appropriately.

Here are the five key principles to promote well-being within long-term care facilities' populations of residents with memory impairments and/or Alzheimer's disease. These principles are:

1) Person-Centered: Care based on the person, their likes, dislikes, hopes, and dreams;
2) Strength-Based: Care based on what a person can do, not on what they cannot do or what disease they have;
3) Recovery-Based: Living each day to the best of their abilities;
4) Meeting Needs: All behavior is a form of communication; and
5) Group Programming: Skill-based groups that give the resident the skills they may need.

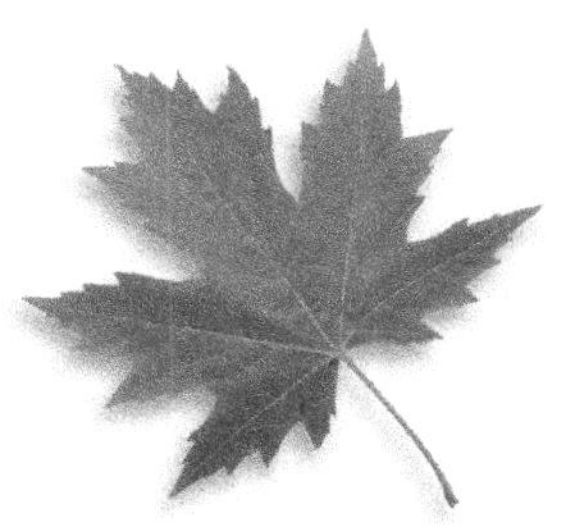

CHAPTER 33

Issues to Remember in Making Care Plans in A Long-Term Care Facility for Individuals With Dementia and/or Alzheimer's Disease

The person with Alzheimer's disease will have difficulty caring for himself/herself and will depend on the facility personnel for assistance. A resident may be willing and able to take their bath one day, and not the next. This does not indicate that the individuals are being mean, stubborn, or manipulative; because of the disease, they may have reduced ability to remember old skills and may have no control over certain behaviors. Some Alzheimer's residents can do some tasks very well, but will need complete assistance with others. The facility leadership team must continuously evaluate each task to determine what the resident can still do.

The most common mistake I see caregivers make is assuming that the residents needs help, simply because they are slow to respond or do the task poorly. The challenge is to give the residents only as much assistance as they need to support their remaining abilities, and to provide structure so that they feel safe and comfortable. A safe and peaceful environment can work miracles on individuals with behavior problems.

The facility leadership and management team must know the residents. In working with each individual in the facility, they should be able to answer the questions listed below to all family members at any given time:

What can the resident do? Examples:

1. Walk without assistance
2. Simple crafts, activities
3. Communicate
    a. With help
    b. Without help

What does the resident need help with? Examples:

1. Impulse control (screaming, biting, combative behavior etc.)
2. Using the bathroom (be specific, i.e., getting his trousers unbuttoned)
3. Dressing (be specific, i.e., patient can put on shirt and trousers but needs assistance with buttons, zipper, etc.)

What are the facility goals for the resident? Examples:

1. Use remaining skills (be specific, i.e., resident draws well, so goal is to maintain this interest and skill as long as possible).

2. Provide safety for person who wanders and tries to leave the facility; also, meet the need for wandering.
3. Maintain the patient's high self-esteem (i.e., provide opportunities in which he experiences success or sense of accomplishment).

A good care plan is one in which the caregiver continuously monitors the changing needs of the person with Alzheimer's disease. It is one which neither demands too much nor too little of the person. It is all about proper balance.

A good care plan is responsive to the unpredictable behaviors of your loved one. The most effective tool in caring for the person with Alzheimer's disease is the facility staff's ability and training, and the professional resources to correctly address problems, situations, or needs, utilizing an appropriate strategy.

Most importantly, because of the unique nature of Alzheimer's disease and related dementia disorders, success often depends on flexibility, creativity, teamwork, and the willingness of the facility staff and the medical team to try different approaches. What works today may not work tomorrow.

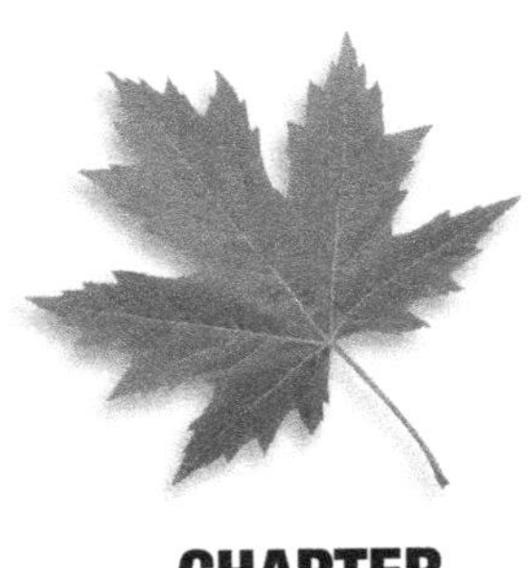

CHAPTER 34

Ten Mistakes People Make When Choosing a Long-Term Care Facility

When families and seniors select a long-term care community, it is a momentous, life-changing decision. You want to get it right the first time. It can be such an intimidating choice that many families come down with "analysis paralysis" and indefinitely postpone a decision out of fear of making the wrong choice. Fortunately, the decision becomes easier as you expand your knowledge. Here are ten common mistakes that families make during the process of selecting a senior community:

1. Not Being Realistic About Current or Future Needs

It is important to balance optimism with a dose of realism. Be realistic about you or your loved one's current care needs as well as their anticipated care needs. Ideally, you will choose a community that is equipped to provide care now, and in the future as your loved one ages. For example, if your loved one has Alzheimer's disease, it may be prudent to choose a community where dedicated memory care is available, even if it is not necessary at the moment. Moving a loved one from facility to facility is not only burdensome and costly on the long-term financial planning to your family, it can also be emotionally and physically detrimental to the senior, particularly a loved one who is affected by dementia, which makes adapting to changes especially difficult.

2. Judging the Book by its Cover

People, not facilities, provide care. Lavish features are not necessarily an indicator of quality care. Sometimes families assume a community is right for their loved one because it has a high price and lavish features, but later they realize fancy furniture and beautiful landscaping are not telltale indicators of quality care. They often find that they need to move their loved one to another community, one that is, perhaps, less shiny but more appropriate in terms of care or atmosphere. Luxury senior living does not necessarily equate to quality senior care. A beautiful, modern, and upscale facility is just as prone to oversights and errors as a community that looks a little dated or tired, or that has more modest features and amenities than its opulent competitor. Quality of care is not something you can discern just by driving past a community to see how green the lawn is, or by poking your head through the lobby door to gauge the ambiance and whether or not it smells nice. Yes, comfort is important and some seniors appreciate a posh lifestyle, but try to look beyond the overstuffed pillows and other trappings of luxury to get a more balanced view of communities that you are considering.

3. Choosing a Community to Match Your Tastes Instead of the Patient's

Often the adult child chooses the place that they like most instead of thinking about what their loved one likes—for example, new chandeliers and a wonderful heated pool when Mom's house is homey and she never liked swimming. Obviously, we encourage families to get their older loved ones as involved as possible in the decision-making process, but if your loved one is too frail or too afflicted with memory loss to participate in the decision-making process, or to visit communities with you, carefully consider his or her personality and preferences rather than your own as you weigh the options.

4. Overplaying the Importance of Proximity

Another mistake that families make is overemphasizing the importance of finding the closest community possible. Sometimes the adult child chooses the nearest community based on the intention of visiting their parent every day, even though another community 10 or 15 miles further away may be a much better fit. Remember that your parent will be engaged in many activities at the community, and that visiting every day is usually an unrealistic expectation to put on yourself. Go with the best fit.

5. Making a Decision Too Quickly

In the introduction, we noted that some families become so overwhelmed with the decision they need to make that they don't make a decision at all. The opposite can also be true. They are in such a rush to resolve a difficult crisis that they choose the very first open room they find in the very first facility they visit, which is probably even less effective than choosing randomly (for example, the room may be vacant for a reason). While delaying necessary care is obviously dangerous, choosing too quickly is also problematic.

6. Choosing a Community Appropriate for the Patient of Yesteryear Instead of the Patient of Today

The problem with many well-intentioned family plans is that they are making arrangements for the mom that they used to know, and not who she has become. For instance, it would be misguided for a family to choose a golf-oriented senior community for a father who loved the game when he was younger but now has Alzheimer's and arthritis and has not played the game in years.

7. Not Reading the Fine Print

Facility contracts are generally relatively straightforward, at least compared to other kinds of legal documents; but they can still contain confusing legalese, or involve additional fees that are not completely apparent. Some families are caught off guard by fees or price increases that they would have been aware of had they reviewed their contract more carefully. Some communities charge individually for each service ("*à la carte* pricing") while other communities may rank the level of care that a resident needs on a scale (for example, a 1 to 5 scale), with care costs based on the level of care the nursing staff determines is needed. Some communities don't charge a care fee at all, but instead opt to provide an "all inclusive" pricing model, whereby resident fees do not depend at all on care needed. At a community with all inclusive pricing, a very frail resident who requires a high level of care has the same fees as a resident who is mostly or even entirely independent (assuming they are in comparably priced apartments).

8. Going It Alone

There is no need to struggle through the search alone, risking costly mistakes or dangerous blunders.

Many people pride themselves on their independent spirit, but when making a decision this big, it is usually wise to gather multiple perspectives on your senior housing options. Get feedback from as many people as possible: friends who have gone through the process, your care management team of loved ones, a geriatric care manager, and a Senior Living Advisor. This kind of professional can help save you hours of time and stress by narrowing your choices to the places that meet your specific needs. They help families evaluate issues such as care requirements, finances, and amenity preferences.

If you do find that your loved one is living in an inappropriate senior community, don't be afraid to admit that you may have made the wrong decision. Make a change quickly, rather than digging into a situation that is not going to work out in the long run.

9. Fail to Interview

Many family members do not ask for references. Ask to

speak with current residents and/or their responsible party. You will be able to get the real picture of a life at the community.

Ask to review the most recent state survey and talk with the facility licensing agency. In most states it is a public record.

Contact the Ombudsman office representative who is in charge of the facility. Most Ombudsman programs visit each facility on a regular base, sometimes on a weekly base. They can provide you with insight as well (see Chapter 42).

10. Long-Term Financial Planning

Always think about the end game. Many consumers are moving into assisted living; when personal funds are depleted, they are then asked to leave the community. Make sure that the facility you choose has a plan in place to ensure that your loved one will be able to stay at the facility, even if all personal funds have been depleted.

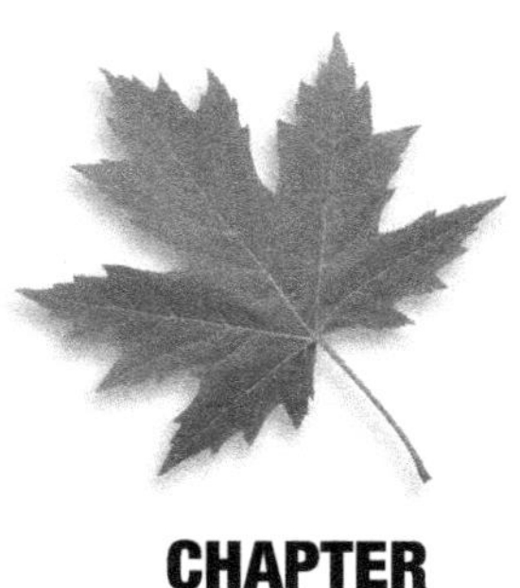

CHAPTER 35

Medication Errors During Care Transition: A Practical Guide for the Caregiver(s)

During an episode of illness, older patients may receive care in multiple settings, placing them at risk for fragmented care and poorly-executed care transitions. For instance, in the course of an episode of illness, a patient may interact with nurses, therapists, and physicians in a hospital, skilled nursing facility, assisted living or rest home, or in the home in conjunction with a home health agency, and finally, in an ambulatory clinic setting. Care from these different sources is frequently not centralized or coordinated, which can result in care that is fragmented. The negative consequences of fragmented care may include the duplication of services, inappropriate or conflicting care recommendations, medication errors, patient and caregiver confusion and distress, and higher costs of care, due to re-hospitalization and use of the emergency department that might have been prevented via the facilitation of a smooth transition from hospital to home. Often information gets lost even during transfer from the emergency room to the hospital admitting floor.

Ensure that the facility has standardized systems to collect and document information about all current medications in place for each patient, and provide the resulting medication list to the receiving caregiver(s) at each care transition point (admission, transfer, discharge, outpatient visit).

<u>Suggested information to be collected includes:</u>

- A list of prescription and non-prescription (over-the-counter) medications, vitamins, nutritional supplements, potentially interactive food items, herbal preparations, and recreational drugs.
- A record of the dose, frequency, route, and timing of the last dose of all medications. Whenever possible, validate the home medication list with the patient and determine the patient's actual level of compliance with prescribed dosing.
- The source(s) of the patient's medications. As appropriate, involve the patient's community pharmacist(s) or primary care provider(s) in collecting and validating the home medication information.
- The reconciliation of medications (i.e., comparison of the patient's medication list compared to the medications being ordered, to identify omissions, duplications, inconsistencies between the patient's medications and clinical conditions, dosing errors, and potential interactions) within specified time frames.
- A process for updating the list, as new orders are written, to reflect all the patient's current medications, including any self-administered medications brought into the organization by the patient.

- A process for ensuring that, at discharge, the patient's medication list is updated to include all medications the patient will be taking following discharge, including new and continuing medications, and previously discontinued "home" medications that are to be resumed. The list should be communicated to the next provider(s) of care and also be provided to the patient as part of the discharge instructions. Medications not to be continued should ideally be discarded by patients.
- Clear assignment of roles and responsibilities for all steps in the medication reconciliation process to qualified individuals, within a context of shared accountability. Those individuals may include the patient's primary care provider, other physicians, nurses, pharmacists, and other clinicians, as well as the primary caregiver(s). The qualifications of the responsible individuals should be determined by the healthcare organization within the limits of applicable law and regulation.
- Access to relevant information and to pharmacist advice at each step in the reconciliation process, to the extent available.

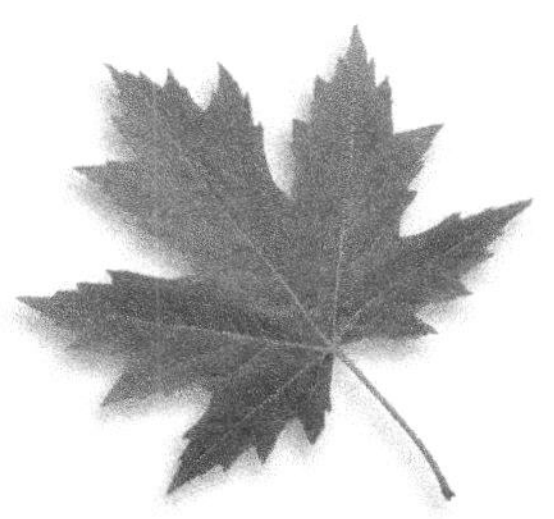

CHAPTER 36

The Newly Admitted Alzheimer's Resident

Families find placement of a loved one in a long-term care facility (Rest Home or Nursing Home) difficult, even in those cases where it is clearly in the best interest of the person and other family members. Invariably, they experience feelings of frustration and a sense of failure at "giving up" care for an impaired loved one. The guilt can be overwhelming. Many caregivers, particularly spouses, experience grief and bereavement over the loss of providing care for the patient at home. This is especially hard when their loved one may feel abandoned, angry, and confused about the placement. It may be difficult to explain the need for the move to the Alzheimer's resident who continually pleads with the family to be taken home. Caregivers may doubt the timing and appropriateness of their decision. They need support, especially if they are being criticized by other family members for placing their relative in a long-term setting.

How well the caregiver copes with the decision will depend on many factors: past relationships, their feelings about caregiving responsibilities, unresolved conflicts within the family, and the support available both before and after placement. Many caregivers overcompensate for feelings of guilt, anxiety, or helplessness by spending an inordinate amount of time in the facility, continuing to help with bathing, dressing, and feeding the loved one, just as they had been doing at home.

Both resident and family will need time to make the adjustment to the placement. Specifically, the resident will need to:

1. "Learn" his place in the facility (i.e., his room, his roommate, the dining room, etc.);
2. Adjust to new and unfamiliar schedules;
3. Cope with a very complex environment, including people he considers strangers or "ill";
4. Trust that staff will not harm him and will care for him.

An established routine and a sense of security will be important for the newly admitted resident. Expect a period of distrust and suspicion. Allow the resident time to get to know the caregivers. Tolerate behaviors which may be reactions to the new environment. Both resident and family may need to express grief, anger, or sadness about changes they can do nothing about.

Let families share their knowledge and experience about their relative. Many of the behavior problems associated with Alzheimer's disease were very likely noticeable at home. The caregiver may be able to offer "unique solutions" to the problems, even suggesting ways to prevent problem situations from occurring. Additionally, let the family share a bit of their relative's history and personality, which will address their need to preserve his dignity, past accomplishments, and history of being a productive, competent person.

Caregivers, especially spouses, may need help in resolving feelings about old promises: "I will never put you in a nursing home." Remind the individual that the resident's needs are very different now than when that promise was made, because the resident is now a very different person. Families may need to be reminded of the very positive aspects of the facility care.

Finally, families need the assurance that staff will view their loved one not just as debilitated and dependent, but as one who can benefit from individualized attention; and that the staff will recognize the opportunity to support the resident in completing a task, no matter how long it takes or how imperfect the job. The resident's increase in self-esteem will be ample reward for him and his family.

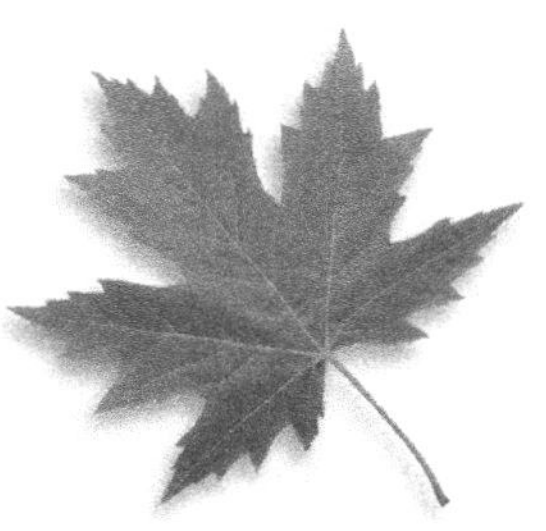

CHAPTER 37

Helping Families Adjust After Placement of a Loved One in a Long-Term Care Facility

Family members confronted with the difficult decision of whether to place a resident with Alzheimer's disease into an institution, find it helpful to have explicit criteria on which to base their decision. Regular incontinence of bladder and bowel, inability of the patient to cooperate in his or her care, inability of the patient to realize that he or she is at home with familiar caregivers, the withdrawal of a paid caregiver, risk to the health of the primary caregiver, and primary caregiver burnout are all grounds for considering institutional placement. Options include rest homes and nursing homes with dementia-specific programs. Institution-like care can be provided at home, but this is expensive, and may be inconvenient and stressful for family members. Hospice care is appropriate at the end of the resident's life.

As a normal response, families confronted with Alzheimer's disease may progress through five stages of adjustment: denial, over-involvement, anger, guilt, and acceptance. These responses may occur independently of one another and not necessarily in the following order.

Denial. The initial response is often that nothing is wrong. Denial can also reappear as false hopes that treatment will cure the patient. Information about the disease can help families understand what is happening, and what to expect.

Over-involvement. The responsible family member attempts to compensate for the illness and its impairments. While being over-involved in the resident's care, the caregiver may refuse assistance from staff, reject advice from the staff, and as a result, feel isolated. Sometimes the primary caregiver will try to meet every need of the patient, even though it is not realistic to do so. The caregiver needs to feel welcome at the facility, and be encouraged to participate in facility activities, programs, and meals, to build a level of confidence in the facility staff.

Anger. Anger can occur when the family realizes that attempts at compensation have failed, and physical and emotional burdens begin to take their toll. Long-standing and interpersonal problems and unresolved issues can be troubling at this stage, if the root of the anger is not addressed. Support groups can help family members work through their feelings of anger, and the other families in the group can offer empathy, having gone through the same process themselves. If anger becomes severe, family members may need to be encouraged to enter counseling, so that hostility does not stand in the way of patient care or sever important family ties. The facility staff needs to provide to the family members accurate, current reports on the emotional and physical condition of their loved one.

Guilt. Guilt is often experienced when the resident can no longer be cared for at home and instead must be placed in a rest home or nursing home facility. Unresolved feelings of anger or guilt can lead to depression. These feelings are normal responses to extreme stress, and should be recognized as such. It is what caregivers and family members then do to resolve their feelings that really makes a difference, and this is where the facility staff needs to support them the most.

Acceptance. At some point, the family will reach resolution or acceptance of the problems. Acceptance comes from a full understanding of the disease and its effect on the family, as well as from recognizing that the loved one is adjusting well to the new setting. Support, education, and other resources can help families move toward acceptance, and must be provided throughout the duration of placement.

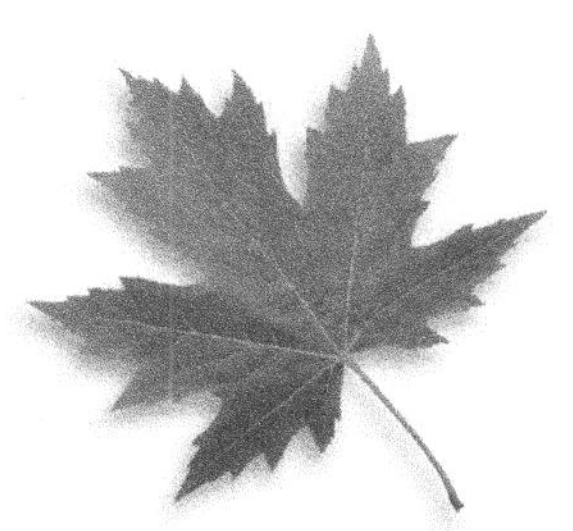

CHAPTER 38

The Resident's Education Program

An education program specifically for residents and family members should include the principles of "Choice, Dignity, and Individuality" to help the resident maintain independence and quality of life to the greatest extent possible. Key points to be integrated are as follows:

- Lifestyle changes that can decrease incontinence and voiding symptoms
- Self-toileting programs
- Identification of products that can manage urine leakage, maintain skin integrity, and increase activity (supplies are usually covered by insurance)
    - Absorbent products
    - Disposables
    - Reusable products
    - Perineal care: excellent peri care is recommended with each change

- Skin barriers and care ointment
- External catheters for men: Texas catheter with secure method of application
- Intermittent catheterization, with a doctor's recommendation and order
- Pelvic organ support devices

• Framing of attitudes

- Help residents and their families understand that incontinence is not necessarily a normal part of aging.
- Inform residents and their family members of the variety of approaches to maintain continence. When one approach is not successful, there are others that might be more advantageous.
- Encourage residents to share with caregivers:
    - Their efforts to maintain continence;
    - Their frustrations when coping with incontinence;
    - Their successes and their appreciation of staff support.

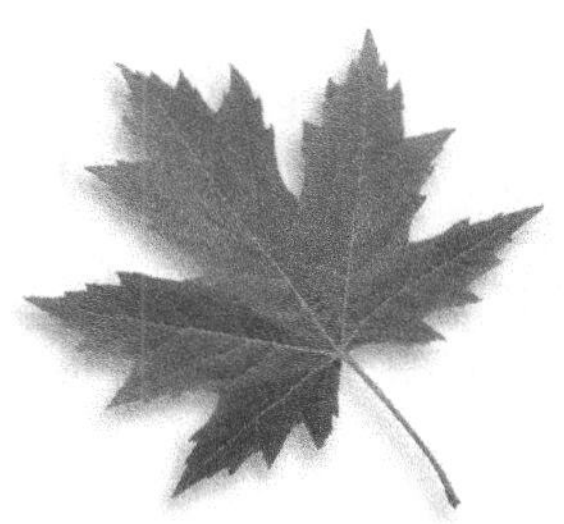

CHAPTER 39

Benefits of a Continence Care Program

for Individuals With Memory Impairment and Alzheimer's Disease in a Long-Term Care Setting

Resident incontinence represents a major challenge for the long-term care (LTC) industry. It negatively impacts residents on many levels and has a significant economic impact on the service provider, both in terms of the support care required and direct-expense costs.

Urinary incontinence (UI) is defined as the complaint of any involuntary leakage of urine. In LTC facilities, more than 50 percent of persons experience UI either occasionally or on a regular basis, and many would argue that the rate is even higher. UI is a contributing factor to skin breakdown, falls, urinary tract infections, social isolation, frustration, anxiety, calling out, and wandering.

Key Facts

- One in three women has some form of incontinence.

- It is estimated that 5-15 percent of those with urinary incontinence also have fecal incontinence.
- A National Association for Continence survey of its members indicated that 16 percent of all those who were 75 years or older admitted that their incontinence had not been diagnosed by a healthcare professional.

A Continence Care Program brings numerous benefits to long-term care communities and to individuals with memory impairment. Education and behavioral changes increase the likelihood that residents can maintain continence, regain continence, or lessen the severity of incontinence. Those residents who are considered at highest risk of developing incontinence are given tools for maintaining control, while others gain new freedoms by addressing reversible factors that may have induced incontinence. Even those with persistent incontinence can learn ways of effectively treating or managing incontinence.

Resident Benefits:

- Improved quality of life, with a greater sense of independence and self-sufficiency;
- Fewer transfers between hospitals and the place of residence;
- Lengthier stays in assisted living with the opportunity to age in place;
- Fewer complications and a reduction in morbidity factors that are indirectly associated with incontinence, such as falls and fractures, dehydration, and urinary tract infections.

Long-Term Care Community Benefits:

- Retain residents in one facility for longer periods of time, by postponing or eliminating the need for nursing home transfers that result from persistent or unmanageable incontinence (some facilities will not keep patients who have unmanageable incontinence issues);
- Improve staff morale through training that allows the facility caregivers to play an active role in enabling residents to maintain their continence, to reverse factors causing their incontinence, or to more effectively manage their incontinence.

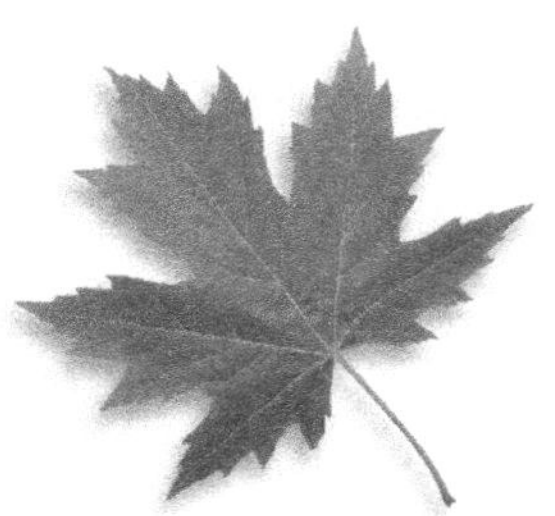

CHAPTER 40

Preservation of Dignity and Quality of Life of the Alzheimer's Resident

The concept of dignity is subjective, and may have different meanings for each person. It is beneficial to have an understanding of what the resident was like before the illness. Remember that several aspects of individuality must be met:

- The identity of the person: how does he or she wish to be addressed? Is there a title, such as Doctor, that is appropriate?
- Respect for privacy: a person who has always disrobed in private may react negatively to being undressed by a stranger.
- The appearance of the resident: attending to grooming and personal hygiene can improve a resident's self-esteem.
- The resident is an adult: even though cognitive deficits exist, the resident has experienced the joys and challenges of several decades of living. To treat residents as children is inappropriate and demeaning. Using words and touch in

ways that allow them to feel valued as individuals is beneficial. People with Alzheimer's disease still have a need to make contributions and to feel that they have some control over their lives. They are more content when they are encouraged to remain active and involved, utilizing their remaining strengths and abilities.

- Physical and psychological comfort: people with Alzheimer's disease have the same basic needs that healthy individuals have. Unmet needs will be reflected in the resident's behavior. The behavior will not change as long as the need remains unmet. Meeting physical needs can prevent discomfort related to hunger, thirst, restlessness, constipation, or the desire to void.
- When people do not feel safe they become anxious: if residents feel threatened, they may strike out verbally or physically. Persons with Alzheimer's disease may feel unsafe much of the time, because they do not understand the environment and what is going on around them.
- People with Alzheimer's disease also need to love and be loved: they should be touched, be hugged, and have eye contact with caregivers. Care providers should converse with them on their level without being condescending, should compliment them on their appearance, and should provide quiet, private areas for visits. Spouses should know that it is acceptable to express affection.
- It is useful to plan activities compatible to the abilities of each individual: each person needs the opportunity to experience a feeling of success.
- Caregivers should listen to the resident: what is expressed

may not sound rational to others, but it does to the person who is speaking.

Family and staff should consider the wishes of the resident before initiating a treatment that may prove to be more harmful than beneficial. For example, starting an IV for feeding or for administering antibiotics to treat an infection may not be in the best interests of the resident, if he or she must be restrained to prevent dislodging of the needle. Acknowledge the individual's autonomy. When a resident is too demented to make decisions, the family must consider what their loved one would have wanted, rather than what they themselves want.

Be honest with Alzheimer's disease residents, while still being optimistic, when answering their questions. Let them know that although the disease is progressive and there is no cure, there are still treatment options. Honesty from caregivers often encourages residents to consider the future, and to make decisions about their future care as their condition worsens.

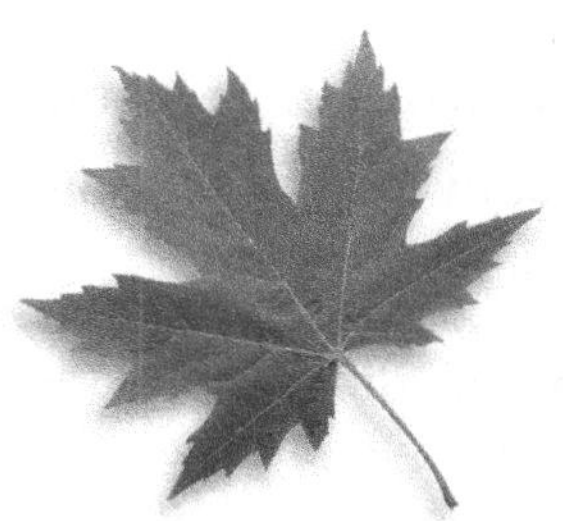

CHAPTER 41

Long-Term Care Facilities: Navigating the Levels of Care

Nearly half of all Americans will need long-term care at some point in their lives. In fact, one in five over the age of 50 is at a high risk of needing long-term care within the next 12 months. Therefore, planning is crucial if you are to designate a facility that will be able to provide your loved one, relative, or friend with the highest quality of care and life in a safe and secure environment. Having a safe and secure environment helps to diminish the feeling of loss or guilt that some people experience when entering or placing a loved one in a long-term care facility. Additionally, the right environment aids in making the transition less stressful for the new resident, family, and loved ones.

Making the decision to reside in a long-term care setting can be a difficult one to make. The best scenario is one where all parties realistically evaluate both the current situation and how it may change in the short- and long-term future. Ideally, being proactive will help everyone arrive at a mutual decision that is the best for all parties involved. The first step in the planning process is having the conversation about a person's long-term care wishes.

The long-term care facility placement options in your state will include some or all of these levels: senior housing, independent living, assisted living, rest home facility (residential care facility), and nursing home.

When trying to navigate through the different levels of care options, there are specific criteria that should be considered. It is important that you check these aspects of a care facility or service in person. Visit facilities and observe carefully. Ask yourself the following questions:

Finances. How much does the facility cost? Does the facility accept Medicaid after personal funds are depleted or private long-term care insurance? Is the facility approved by insurance as a long-term care provider? How much can your family afford in regard to long-term care? What is the "look-back" on the state and federal level? The look-back period is the five-year period immediately preceding the application to qualify for nursing home Medicaid benefits (the Nursing Home period is five years and the Rest Home is only one year). Gifts made prior to this period do not affect a person's eligibility for Medicaid.

In order to be eligible to receive Medicaid coverage while in a nursing home, an individual must have very limited resources. Certain assets, such as the home and retirement accounts, may be exempt in some circumstances.

Gifts made by an individual during the five-year Medicaid look-back period will generally disqualify that person for nursing home Medicaid benefits for a period of time based on the dollar value of the gifts made. So, the larger the gift, the longer the penalty period will be before eligibility is met. In other words, an individual cannot simply give away assets as gifts and then claim to have limited resources, thereby qualifying for Medicaid coverage.

If the person applying for residence in a nursing home is the beneficiary of a trust, the placement of the money in that trust is treated as a gift and subject to the look-back rules, if the trust is irrevocable. Irrevocable means that the assets in the trust cannot be returned for any reason to the person who funded the trust.

Will the facility allow your loved one to stay once all personal funds have been depleted?

Expertise. Is the facility equipped to care for people with memory impairment or Alzheimer's disease and related conditions? Are staff members trained to handle behavioral issues such as aggression and wandering? Is the staff physician familiar with Alzheimer's-related healthcare issues? How many residents with similar health challenges are living in the facility at any given time?

Compliance Records with State and Federal Regulatory Agencies. Check the facility record and most recent survey. It is a public record. Is the facility compliant with all regulations? Contact the Ombudsman office as well (see Chapter 42). They can be a great resource.

Day-to-Day Care. How do staff members interact with the residents? Does the facility have a friendly atmosphere? Is it too noisy or chaotic? What kinds of activities and social opportunities are available for people with Alzheimer's disease? Check staff-to-patient ratios for both the nursing and activity departments.

Physical Environment. Does the physical layout of the facility provide opportunities for socializing as well as privacy? Is the facility clean, bright, safe, and secure?

Management. What was your gut feeling after the interview with management? How easy (or difficult) might it be to discuss potential concerns with them? Does management have an open door policy to talk with clients?

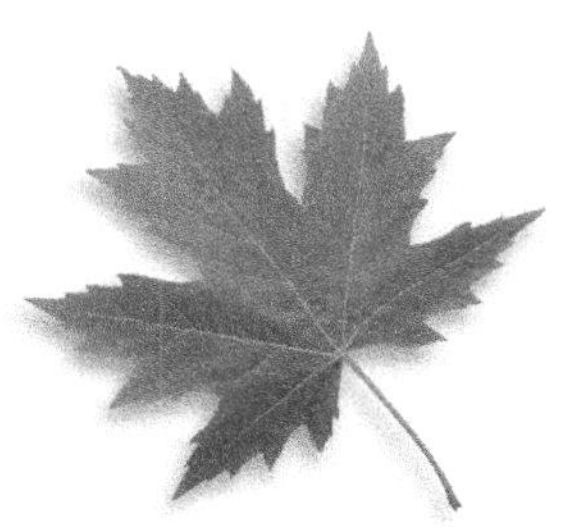

CHAPTER 42

Long-Term Care Ombudsman Program

What Is The Office of Ombudsman for Long-Term Care?

The Ombudsman office advocates for person-directed living throughout the health care continuum, a policy which respects individual values and preferences, and preserves individual rights.

Regional ombudsmen and volunteers work with consumers, citizens, nursing homes, rest homes, hospitals, assisted living facilities, home care providers, social service agencies, and public agencies to enhance the quality of life and services for individuals receiving healthcare and supportive services at home, in hospitals, in nursing homes, in residential care facilities (rest homes), boarding care homes, and in other community settings, such as housing with services (assisted living, customized living), adult foster care, and adult day centers.

The Ombudsman Office also works to enhance the quality of life and services for consumers by advocating for reform in the healthcare and social services delivery systems through changes in state and federal law and administrative policy.

What Is An Ombudsman?

An Ombudsman is an independent consumer advocate. Ombudsmen investigate complaints concerning the health, safety, welfare, and rights of long-term care consumers; they work to resolve individual concerns; they also identify problems and advocate for changes to address those problems, at no charge to the consumer. Ombudsmen also offer information and consultation about nursing homes, boarding care homes, housing with services, assisted living, customized living, home care, and hospital services, rights, and regulations. Additionally, ombudsmen work with providers of long-term care services to promote a culture of person-directed living.

Who Do Ombudsman Serve?

- Residents of nursing homes and boarding care homes
- Residents of other adult care homes (i.e., housing with services, assisted living, customized living or foster care)
- Persons receiving home care services
- Medicare beneficiaries with hospital access or discharge concerns
- Anyone seeking consultation about long-term care services

How Can They Help?

Ombudsmen provide information and consultation about consumer rights and the regulations that apply to long-term care facilities, home and community-based settings, and home care services.

Ombudsmen help to resolve disputes between consumers and providers of long-term care services, regardless of where those services are provided.

Ombudsmen handle complaints and problems relating to:

- Quality care/services
- Quality of life
- Rights violations
- Access to services
- Service termination
- Discharge or eviction
- Public benefit programs

You can request a variety of consumer resources using the Consumer Resources Order Form (http://www.voycestl.org/files/7013/7722/9844/Directory_OrderForm_Website_PDF_file_for_website.pdf).

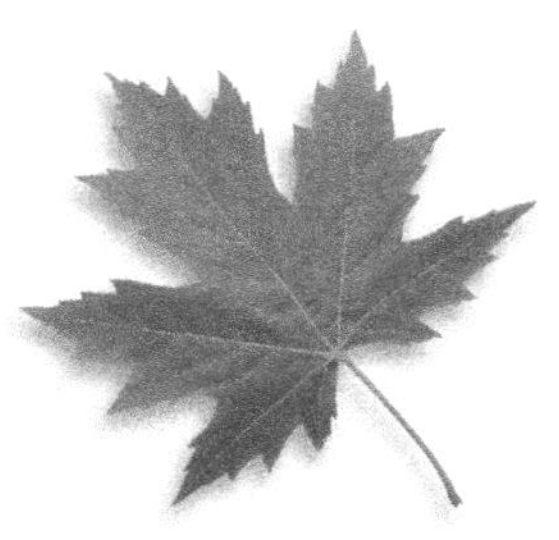

CHAPTER 43

Long-Term Care Facility Selection Checklist

This checklist can serve as a useful tool when investigating and evaluating nursing homes, rest homes, residential care facilities, and assisted living facilities. The checklist is divided into two sections: 1) Quality Dimensions and 2) Practical Dimensions.

Although the quality dimensions are crucial, they need to be balanced by practical considerations. Sometimes the best home might be a little further from your home than you had hoped to drive. But if this facility provides the best possible care for your loved one, it will be worth a visit. Depending on the person's needs and preferences, some questions can be more important than others.

Keep in mind the following general tips:

- Start the process early, before there is a crisis.
- Involve the prospective resident as much as possible in the process, if this is possible and practical.

- Use the checklist to get an overall impression of the facility and its practices.
- Pay special attention to how residents are being treated by staff, and the quality and responsiveness of the services.
- Don't be sold only on the attractiveness of the facility. The care provided is the most vital element of the placement.
- Narrow the options down to two or three facilities.
- Visit each facility several times. Show up without notice. When you visit, walk through the entire facility, and visit at different times of the day: visit at night and/or on the weekend.
- Make sure you visit during a mealtime.
- Obtain a copy of the admission agreement. Read it carefully. Understand the services, costs, and conditions for transfer. Always look for the availability of all-inclusive care. Knowing the monthly cost of care in advance allows for the best financial planning practices.
- Before you make a final decision, check the latest annual survey report and any citations issued by the state licensing agency. Facilities should make these reports available to you upon request. Talk with current residents and, if possible, their family members.

Quality Dimensions

Quality of Care and Service

[ ] Do residents appear well cared for?

[ ] Are residents up, clean, and dressed by 8:30 a.m.?

[ ] Are the residents well groomed (e.g., shaved, clean clothes, nails trimmed, and hair combed)?

[ ] Is there a written plan of care for each resident? How often is the care plan reviewed and updated? By whom?

[ ] Does the facility offer programs and/or services that meet your particular care needs (e.g., dementia)?

[ ] What is the system for distribution of medications? Does the facility's licensing permit include dispensing of medications? Or does it only permit the facility to remind the resident to take his or her medications? Who actually dispenses meds? What is their level of training?

[ ] Is there a medical director and/or physician(s) on premises?

[ ] Is a mental health director (physician) available?

[ ] Does the facility provide transportation to medical services? Does it charge for this kind of transportation?

[ ] Are there clear procedures for responding to medical emergencies?

Quality of Food

[ ] Does the food look and smell appealing? Are fresh ingredients used?

[ ] Do residents seem to be enjoying the food?

[ ] Does the facility offer two substantial meals, lunch and dinner, or is dinner a smaller meal? Unfortunately, many facilities provide only sandwiches for dinner.

[ ] Are residents receiving needed dining assistance?

[ ] Are foods served at appropriate temperatures?

[ ] Do menus offer daily choices? How often are menus changed? Ask to see a copy of the week's menu.

[ ] Can the facility meet special dietary needs and ethnic preferences?

[ ] Are nutritious snacks available?

[ ] Is fresh drinking water readily available?

[ ] Is a staff dietician available to review residents' dietary needs and provide recommendations?

[ ] Does the facility make provisions to serve residents in their rooms when needed? Is there an extra cost for this?

Quality of Social Interaction

[ ] Are residents interacting with staff and/or each other?

[ ] Are residents engaged in meaningful activities?

[ ] Does the facility have a planned activities program? Are activity calendars posted? What activities are provided on weekends?

[ ] Is there a designated staff member who coordinates activities? Are activities individualized, or only conducted in large groups?

[ ] Do volunteers and outside groups regularly visit the facility?

[ ] Are there planned trips outside the facility?

[ ] Is transportation provided for shopping and personal errands? Are there extra fees for this?

[ ] Are pets permitted? Does the facility have its own pets?

[ ] Are residents encouraged to bring in some of their own furnishings?

[ ] Are religious services offered at the facility?

Quality of Participation

[ ] Are residents and family members involved in assessment and care planning?

[ ] Do residents have an opportunity to provide input into menu and activity planning?

[ ] Are there procedures for responding to requests for information and complaints?

[ ] Are the Ombudsman Program's poster and telephone number posted?

[ ] Does the facility have a residents' council? Does the facility have a family council or support group?

Quality of Staff

[ ] How long has the key staff been working at the facility (i.e., administrator, director of nursing, activities director, head chef, floor manager, nurse consultant, medical director)?

[ ] Has there been major turnover in key staff recently?

[ ] How many direct-care staff are there for each shift?

[ ] What is the staff-to-resident ratio? What is the ratio on the night shift? Weekends?

[ ] How many hours of nursing care per day are available?

[ ] What is the turnover rate among direct-care staff?

[ ] Does the direct-care staff understand and speak English?

[ ] What special training does the staff receive in working with individuals with dementia?

[ ] Do the administration and staff members know the residents by name?

[ ] Does the staff take time to talk with residents?

[ ] Do members of the administration and staff interact with residents in a respectful way?

[ ] How long does it take for staff to respond to a resident's request for help or to the call bell?

[ ] Does the staff respect residents' privacy by knocking on doors or announcing themselves before entering rooms?

[ ] Does the staff wear name badges?

Quality of the Environment

[ ] Are emergency exit signs prominently posted and lit?

[ ] Is the overall decor pleasant and homelike?

[ ] Is the environment clean and odor-free?

[ ] Is the facility quiet or noisy?

[ ] Is the temperature comfortable?

[ ] Does the building seem safe and free from dangerous hazards? Is it cluttered?

[ ] Are the residents' rooms, hallways, and common areas well lit?

[ ] Are floors finished with non-skid material? Are carpets firm and safe, able to provide for easy walking and designed to prevent falls?

[ ] Is the dining room pleasant and inviting?

[ ] Are common areas, bedrooms, and bathrooms accessible to wheelchairs and walkers?

[ ] Are bathrooms conveniently located?

[ ] Do all bathrooms, showers, and bathtubs have handgrips or rails?

[ ] Are call signals easily accessible to residents? At bedside? In bathrooms?

[ ] Do residents' rooms offer privacy, especially in shared rooms?

[ ] Is there a convenient place to conduct private conversation?

[ ] Does every resident's room include for each occupant a bedside table, reading light, chest of drawers, and at least one comfortable chair?

[ ] Is there adequate storage space for clothing and personal belongings in each room?

[ ] Does the facility have extra storage space for residents' belongings?

[ ] Are there outside sitting or walking areas for residents? Are any of them covered to protect the residents from sun and rain?

[ ] Is there a fenced yard? Is it secured?

[ ] Is a disaster plan posted? How often does the facility hold drills?

Practical Dimensions

Accessibility

[ ] Is the facility located close to the family and friends who will be visiting most frequently?

[ ] Are you willing to drive a little longer for a well-established facility?

[ ] Is the facility near public transportation?

[ ] Is the facility in a location that is safe to visit at night?

[ ] Is the facility convenient to the resident's doctor? Home health agency?

[ ] Is the facility close to a hospital?

[ ] Are families and friends welcome at any time, or are there strict visiting hours?

[ ] Are emergency services, such as fire and police stations, close by?

Suitability

[ ] Does the facility have a good reputation in the community?

[ ] Will the facility provide a list of references?

[ ] Are residents and/or family members willing to talk with you about the facility?

[ ] How does the staff treat you when you visit?

[ ] Did they answer all your questions to your satisfaction?

[ ] Did they show you around the entire facility? Were any areas or sections not shown to you? Why?

[ ] Do you feel that the staff consists of people you can work with and communicate with honestly?

[ ] How would you or your loved one fit in? Is this facility compatible with your lifestyle?

[ ] Can you imagine yourself or your loved one living here?

[ ] What was your overall impression of the facility when you visited?

Affordability

[ ] Are there any upfront fees (e.g., assessment, community fees)?

[ ] What services are not included in the basic rate?

[ ] What is the cost for extra services? For different levels of care? How is the need for extra services or higher levels of care determined?

[ ] What are the costs for specialized services (e.g., dementia care)?

[ ] Are the costs and payment schedule clearly described in the admission agreement?

[ ] Are the total monthly charges affordable over time?

[ ] Would your loved one be able to continue living there after all personal funds are depleted?

[ ] Did the facility explain the available emergency aid programs to you?

Pay special attention to the following factors when considering a placement for an individual with dementia.

Environment

[ ] Is the facility calm and quiet?

[ ] Does the facility provide soft music and/or natural scents to create a soothing atmosphere?

[ ] Is the facility well lit? Is there adequate natural light?

[ ] Are there complex patterns on carpets or walls, which can cause confusion or other difficulties?

[ ] Can staff easily observe the facility's common areas? Outside areas?

[ ] Can staff easily observe the residents' rooms?

[ ] How does the environment promote resident functioning (e.g., a picture of a toilet on the bathroom door)?

[ ] Does the facility have a wander-alert system?

[ ] Are the doors equipped with a system to delay exit? The exception, of course, involves an emergency, such as fire.

[ ] Is there a locked or secured outside area for walking?

Philosophy of Care

[ ] Is the facility's philosophy for caring for persons with dementia consistent with your beliefs?

[ ] Does the facility provide services to persons at all stages of the disease process?

[ ] What conditions or behaviors determine whether a facility will admit and retain someone with dementia?

[ ] Is dementia care provided in a separate unit or as an integrated part of facility services?

[ ] Is the facility's philosophy and practice of handling "difficult behaviors" compatible with your views? Offer a few

examples and ask staff how they would handle the situation.

[ ] What is the facility's philosophy in using physical restraints to deal with certain behaviors? Rest home facilities for the elderly are severely restricted by law in the use of restraints and psychoactive medications.

[ ] Does the facility recommend the use of psychoactive drugs to treat behaviors?

Services

[ ] Are there activities specially designed for individuals with dementia?

[ ] Do activity programs operate throughout the day? Evenings? Weekends?

[ ] Are activities individualized for each resident?

[ ] Does the facility provide nutritious snack foods?

[ ] Are water and decaffeinated beverages readily available throughout the day?

[ ] Does the facility conduct periodic night checks?

[ ] How many staff members are awake during the night?

Staff

[ ] Is the assessment and care-planning process coordinated by a person with special knowledge and training in dementia?

[ ] What role does direct-care staff have in the care-planning process?

[ ] What role does the resident and family or legal representative play in the care-planning process?

[ ] Is the activity program planned and coordinated by a person with special training? Is this person full-time? Have assistants?

[ ] Does the activity coordinator design customized activities for each resident? Who leads one-on-one activities?

[ ] Is a staff member assigned to work with the same residents all the time, or do the staff members rotate among residents?

[ ] What is the ratio of direct-care staff to residents in each shift?

[ ] What type of specialized dementia training does the direct-care staff receive initially and on an on-going basis? What is the content? Number of hours of training received? Frequency?

[ ] Specifically, what type of training does the direct-care staff receive in handling difficult behaviors? What is the content? Number of hours of training received? Frequency?

[ ] Who supervises the direct-care staff? What are their qualifications?

[ ] What special training do the administrators and supervisors receive in dementia care? What is the content? Number of hours of training received? Frequency?

Other

[ ] Is the facility in contact with experts in dementia care, such as Alzheimer's diagnostic centers, the Alzheimer's Association, or Regional Caregiver Resource Centers?

[ ] Does the facility have a family support group or does it refer to community-based groups?

[ ] What does the facility charge for special dementia services? Is there a basic rate that covers all services? Are there additional charges for changing care needs?

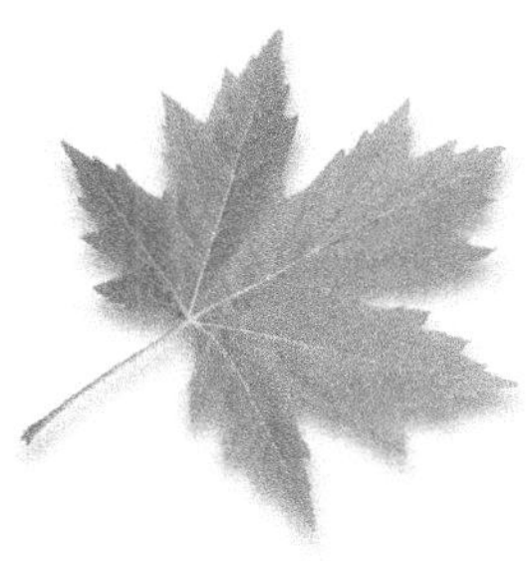

Author's Notes

I set out to write a comprehensive book with a fresh approach for caregivers and family members who are dealing with, and assisting, individuals diagnosed with Alzheimer's disease at any stage of the disease.

This book has been in the making for the past decade. I gathered as much information as I could from my 27-plus years as an administrator of different levels of residential care and rest home facilities that specialized in caring for individuals diagnosed with Alzheimer's disease. In the past couple of years, more new books have come out and some very good research reports have been published by well-known researchers in the Alzheimer's field. This field is moving at a very rapid speed; however, no final solution or remedy is on the immediate horizon for those suffering from dementia and related diseases.

My goals in writing this book are simple. I want to: 1) provide as much information as I can that will assist individuals diagnosed with Alzheimer's and/or other related dementia diseases, 2) make it readable, 3) be brief on each topic without overdoing it or confusing the readers and caregivers, and 4) write it for everyone who wants to learn, and subsequently utilize, my suggestions to form an individualized care plan.

Whether you are a family member, nurse, caregiver, or other professional in the long-term care industry, I hope this book speaks to you.

There is a lot of information to digest, but each chapter represents an essential element of person-centered care, or a special guideline of what to do if a particular situation arises.

It is my hope that if, after reading the book, you now feel differently about the disease and the available tools and resources, then you've already begun the process of getting more help or support, which will place you way ahead of the curve; this is a good thing for you, your loved one(s), and the patient you are caring for.

Take this information and share it with everyone who can benefit from it, and please, put these ideas into action.

Recommended Reading

1. ***Alzheimer's Disease*** organized by Leonardo Caixeta, Brazil, ISBN 8536327006.

2. ***Movement with Meaning: a Multisensory Program for Individuals with Early-Stage Alzheimer's Disease*** by B. Larsen, 2006, ISBN-13: 978-1932529142.

3. ***Let's Look Together: an Interactive Picture Book*** by R. Cebul Ziegler, 2009, ISBN-13: 978-1932529517.

4. ***American Psychiatric Publishing Textbook of Alzheimer's and Other Dementias*** edited by M.F. Weiner and A.M. Lipton, 2009, ISBN 978-1-58562-278-8.

5. ***Mayo Clinic on Alzheimer's Disease*** by R. Peterson, 2002, ISBN-13: 978-1893005228.

6. ***Finding Life in the Land of Alzheimer's: One Daughter's Hopeful Story*** by L. Kessler, 2008, ISBN-13: 978-0143113683.

7. ***Losing my mind: an Intimate Look at Life with Alzheimer's*** by T. DeBaggio, 2003, ISBN-13: 978-0743205665.

8. ***Thousand Mile Stare: One Family's Journey through the Struggle and Science of Alzheimer's*** by G. Reiswig, 2010, ISBN-13: 978-1857885361.

9. ***36 Hour Day*** (4th edition or latest available) by N. Mace and P. Rabins, 2006, ISBN-13: 978-0446610414.

10. ***Alzheimer's early stages: First Steps for Family, Friends and Caregivers*** by D. Kuhn and D. Bennett, 2003, ISBN-13: 978-0897933971.

11. ***Alzheimer's advisor: A Caregiver's Guide to Dealing with the Tough Legal and Practical Issues*** by V. E. James, 2008, ISBN-13: 978-0814409244.

12. ***A Dignified life: The Best Friends Approach to Alzheimer's Care, a Guide for Family Caregivers*** by V. Bell and D. Troxel, 2000, ISBN-13: 978-0757300608.

13. ***Moving a Relative With Memory Loss: A Family Caregiver's Guide*** by L. White and B. Spencer, 2006, ISBN-13: 978-0970760913.

14. ***Navigating the Alzheimer's journey: a Compass for Caregiving*** by C. Bowlby Sifton, 2004, ISBN-13: 978-1932529043.

15. ***Understanding Difficult Behaviors: Some practical suggestions for coping with Alzheimer's Disease and Related Illnesses*** by R. Spence and L. White, 2007, ISBN-13: 978-0978902001.

16. ***Caring for a Person with Alzheimer's Disease: Your Easy-to-Use Guide from the National Institute on Aging***, National Institutes of Health, 2012 download or print, http://www.nia.nih.gov/alzheimers/publication/caring-person-alzheimers-disease.

17. ***End of life: Helping With Comfort and Care***, National Institute on Aging, National Institutes of Health, 2010, download or print, http://www.nia.nih.gov/health/publication/end-life-helping-comfort-and-care.

18. ***Decoding darkness: The Search For The Genetic Causes Of Alzheimer's*** by R. Tanzi, 2001, ISBN-13: 978-0738205267.

19. ***Alzheimer's Action Plan: The Experts' Guide to the Best Diagnosis and Treatment for Memory Problems*** by P. Doraiswamy, L. Gwyther, and T. Adler, 2008, ASIN: B001KK6XYQ.

20. ***Best Friends Approach to Alzheimer's Care*** by V. Bell and D. Troxel, 2002, ISBN-13: 978-1878812353.

21. ***Critical Thinking in Long-Term Care Nursing*** by S. Cohen, 2008, ISBN-13: 978-1601461377.

22. ***The Dementia Care Plan Dictionary,*** a behavior-based care plan idea book by M. Nolta and B. Hall, 2005.

23. ***Developing Support Groups for Individuals with Early Stage Alzheimer's Disease: Planning, Implementation, and Evaluation*** by R. Yale, 1995, ISBN-13: 978-1878812.

24. ***Palliative Care for Advanced Alzheimer's and Dementia: Guidelines and Standards for Evidence-Based Care*** edited by G. Martin and M. Sabbagh, 2010, ISBN-13: 978-0826.

25. ***Guide to the Spiritual Dimension of Care for People with Alzheimer's Disease and Related Dementia: More than Body, Brain and Breath*** by E. Shamy, 2003, ISBN-13: 978-1843101291.

26. ***Between Two Worlds: Special Moments of Alzheimer's & Dementia*** by Ellen P. Young, 2003, ISBN-13: 978-1591021636.

27. Spira. A. et al., **Self-reported Sleep and β-Amyloid Deposition in Community-Dwelling Older Adults.** *JAMA Neurology* 2013, 70[12]:1537.

Additional Online Resources for Specific Topics

CHAPTER 1

Alzheimer's Research Center (http://www.alz.org/research/)

Alzheimer's Disease – History and Description (http://www.best-alzheimers-products.com/alzheimers-disease.html)

Guidelines for Alzheimer's Disease Management, 2010 (http://www.cdph.ca.gov/programs/alzheimers/Documents/professional_GuidelineFullReport.pdf)

About Dementia (http://www.alzheimers.org.uk/site/scripts/documents.php?categoryID=200120)

Depression (https://www.alzheimers.org.uk/site/scripts/services_info.php?serviceID=41)

CHAPTER 2

Dr. Aloysius Alzheimer (http://alzheimers-disease.wikispaces.com/Dr.+Alois+Alzheimer)

Diagnostic Guidelines for Alzheimer's Disease: Frequently Asked Questions for Clinicians (http://www.nia.nih.gov/alzheimers/diagnostic-guidelines-alzheimers-disease-frequently-asked-questions-clinicians)

Artherosclerosis (http://www.medicalnewstoday.com/articles/247837.php)

Pneumonia (http://www.medicalnewstoday.com/articles/151632.php)

Pressure ulcers (http://www.medicalnewstoday.com/articles/173972.php)

CHAPTER 4

Shorter Sleep Duration and Poorer Sleep Quality Linked to Alzheimer's Disease Biomarker; Johns Hopkins School of Medicine Brain Science Institute (http://www.jhsph.edu/news/news-releases/2013/spira-sleep-alzheimer.html).

CHAPTER 5

Medication Side Effects (http://alzheimers.about.com/od/treatmentoptions/a/elder_drugs.htm)

CHAPTER 6

Restlessness and Agitation (http://alzheimers.about.com/od/frustration/a/chal_beh_whatis.htm)

Confusion (http://alzheimers.about.com/od/caregivers/a/orientation.htm)

Anxiety (http://www.ec-online.net/knowledge/articles/caringforthecg.html)

Treating behavioral and psychological symptoms of dementia (http://www.alzheimers.org.uk/site/scripts/documents_info.php?documentID=1191)

CHAPTER 20

Caring for a Person with Dementia (http://www.alzheimers.org.uk/site/scripts/documents.php?categoryID=200343)

CHAPTER 26

Inspiration, perspective and advice for you from family caregivers of loved ones with Alzheimer's, Caregiver's Action Network, (formerly National Family Caregivers Association [NFCA]) (http://caregiveraction.org/resources/).

Coping with Caring (https://www.alzheimers.org.uk/site/scripts/documents.php?categoryID=200358)

Carer Support
(https://www.alzheimers.org.uk/site/scripts/documents_info.php?documentID=546)

CHAPTER 43

Ethnicity and the Experience of Alzheimer's Disease by Christine Kennard, Health Central, January 20, 2009 (http://www.healthcentral.com/alzheimers/c/57548/56301/experience/)

Index

C

D

L

M

N

O

P